W9-BLO-693

ASHTANGA YOGA

FOR WOMEN

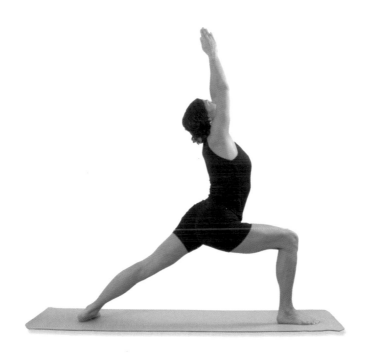

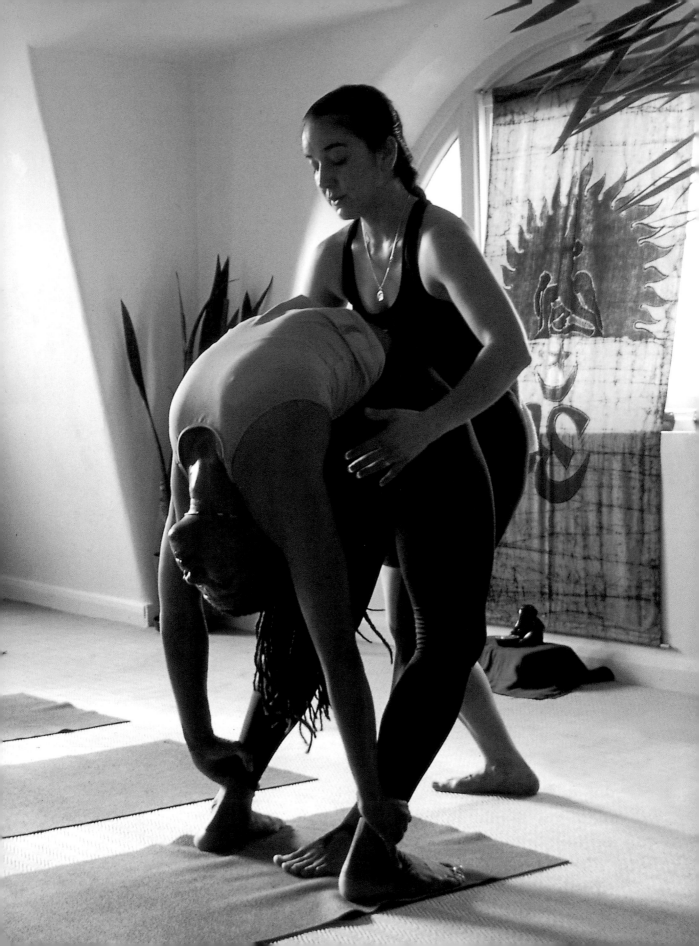

ASHTANGA YOGA
FOR WOMEN

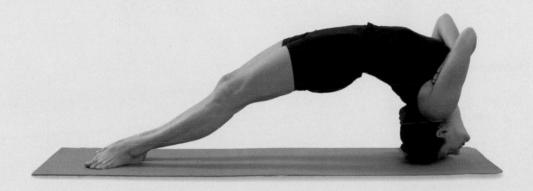

Invigorating mind, body, and spirit with power yoga

Written by Sally Griffyn and Michaela Clarke

Photography by Sally Griffyn

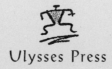

Ulysses Press

This edition first published in the U.S. by Ulysses Press,
P.O. Box 3440, Berkeley, CA 94703
www.ulyssespress.com

ISBN 1-56975-350-4

Library of Congress Control Number 2003100209

First published in Great Britain in 2003 by
Godsfield Press Ltd. wwwgodsfieldpress.com

Copyright © 2003 Godsfield Press Ltd.
Text Copyright © 2003 Sally Griffyn and Michaela Clarke

Designed and produced by The Bridgewater Book Company

All rights reserved. No part of this publication may be
reproduced, stored in a retrieval system or transmitted in any
form, or by any means, electronic, mechanical, photocopying or
otherwise without the prior permission of the publisher.

Sally Griffyn and Michaela Clarke assert the moral right to
be identified as the authors of this work.

Printed and bound in China

10 9 8 7 6 5 4 3 2 1

Distributed in the United States by Publishers Group West
and in Canada by Raincoast Books

Project Designer: Lisa McCormick
Project Editor: Nicola Wright
Picture Researcher: Lynda Marshall

NOTE: Any information given in this book is not
intended to be taken as a replacement for
medical advice. Any person with a condition
requiring medical attention should consult a
qualified medical practitioner or therapist before
beginning any of the postures in this book.

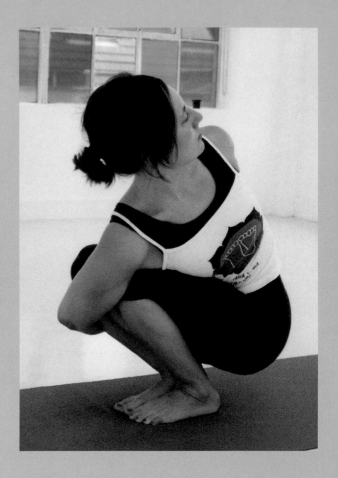

He who binds to himself a joy
Doth the winged life destroy
But he who kisses the joy as it flies,
Lives in Eternity's sunrise.

WILLIAM BLAKE

CONTENTS

INTRODUCTION   6

CHAPTER ONE: INTRODUCTION TO ASHTANGA   8
History of Yoga   10
The Story of Ashtanga   12
What is Ashtanga Vinyasa Yoga?   16

CHAPTER TWO: THE PRIMARY SERIES   20
Preparations for Practice   22
Dancing to the Music of the Breath   23
The Sun Salutations   26
The Standing Postures   34
The Warrior Sequence   56
The Sitting Postures   60
The Finishing Sequence   96
The Breathing Sequence   104

CHAPTER TIIREE: ASHTANGA AND THE CYCLES OF LIFE   106
The Cycles of Life   108
Sun   110
Moon   112
Menstruation   114
Fertility   116
Pregnancy   118
Children and Yoga   120

APPENDIXES
1: Preventing Injuries   122
2: The Yoga of Food   124

USEFUL INFORMATION   126

INDEX   127
Acknowledgments   128

INTRODUCTION

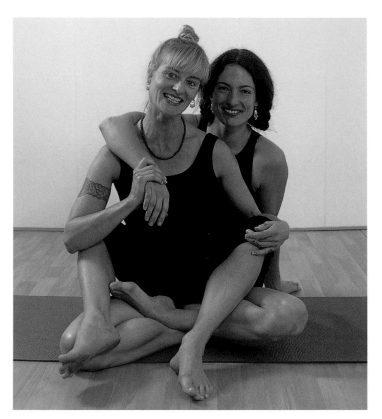

THE AUTHORS, SALLY GRIFFYN (FRONT) AND MICHAELA CLARKE.

This is a book about Ashtanga Yoga and its impact on women. Women have always been part of the Ashtanga community and Sri Krishna Pattabhi Jois (known as Guruji to his devotees), the modern founder of Ashtanga, makes this very clear. He taught his wife Amma and his daughter Saraswati, who now helps him to adjust when he is on tour. Guruji was one of the first to explain the mysteries of Ashtanga to westerners, who first arrived on his doorstep in the 1960s. Women have always practiced this form of yoga alongside men, and Guruji emphasizes that the only prohibitions on a woman's practice are related to the menstrual cycle and pregnancy. Many of Guruji's best and most devoted students are women.

The concept of this book came from conversations we had with women or overheard in the *chai* (tea) stand or changing room, in which women laughed about how difficult it was to do certain asanas with larger breasts, weaker arms, bigger hips, and during pregnancy, and when they simply didn't want to get on the mat for one reason or another.

We also heard about cyclical issues— how their experiences of Ashtanga varied during hard times and good times in their lives. Surprisingly, when times were difficult or they were angry, women often had a good practice, as if the energy moved through and out of them, leaving them more able to cope. Some women interestingly reported different emotional responses at different times of the month. The practice flows like the ebbing and rising of the tides and like the moon, which governs them. Women, who are so intrinsically linked to the moon, move through the cycle, becoming more confident in their Ashtanga practice, and learning over time that everything changes. What was hard becomes easy. Alternatively, one day the postures can feel easy; the next day they may seem impossibly hard. But, with time, the practice deepens, allowing for the layers of personality to be stripped away and subsequently rebuilt.

During our research for this book, we discovered that few women knew how they would need to modify their practice for pregnancy, or why they should not practice certain postures during menstruation. We hope this book offers them useful advice.

The experience of women doing a dynamic yoga practice can be different from that of men because women have different bodies and often different responsibilities in their lives. We hope to address these issues and also offer suggestions that will allow the female body to strengthen safely when practicing yoga.

Ashtanga yoga itself is not specifically designed for men, but is traditionally practiced in India by *Brahmins* (the priestly caste), rather than by workers. It demands the lifestyle that often only a man can have. The disciplinary aspect of the yoga is governed by the implicit idea that a man will have the time to practice for the whole of his life unfettered by childbearing.

Daily discipline is different for women, who are interrupted by time off for menstruation and pregnancy and then childcare. Men who take on childcare to the extent that women have historically, report the same issues arising in their life around having time to practice. In fact, what is discipline for men is consistency of return for women—to return time and time again

to yoga practice in between the demands of lifestyle.

There is also a need for western influences to be understood in relation to this kind of yoga. Ashtanga evolved out of a spiritual path primarily practiced by *sadhus* (Indian holy men), which was then adopted by the privileged members of the household of the maharajah of Mysore. When Guruji decided to devote his life to the practice, he did so in secret, unbeknown to his family. At the time (1927) the attitude in India was much the same as in Europe and the U.S. not that long ago— that those who practiced Ashtanga were on an unusual, alternative spiritual path.

The practice was brought to the west by pioneering students of Guruji in the 1970s. Since then, teachers with a background in other forms of body work have been interpreting the style as taught by Guruji and exchanging information. In many western classes more emphasis is now placed on alignment and strength than would be the case in Mysore where Guruji teaches at the Ashtanga Yoga Research Institute. Some of Guruji's prohibitions, such as only practicing the sequence of asanas in the correct order, and not practicing during menstruation, are sometimes misunderstood.

In this book we hope to honor and respect the teachings of our fondly loved Guruji. We are also excited to represent the knowledge and contributions of teachers in the West.

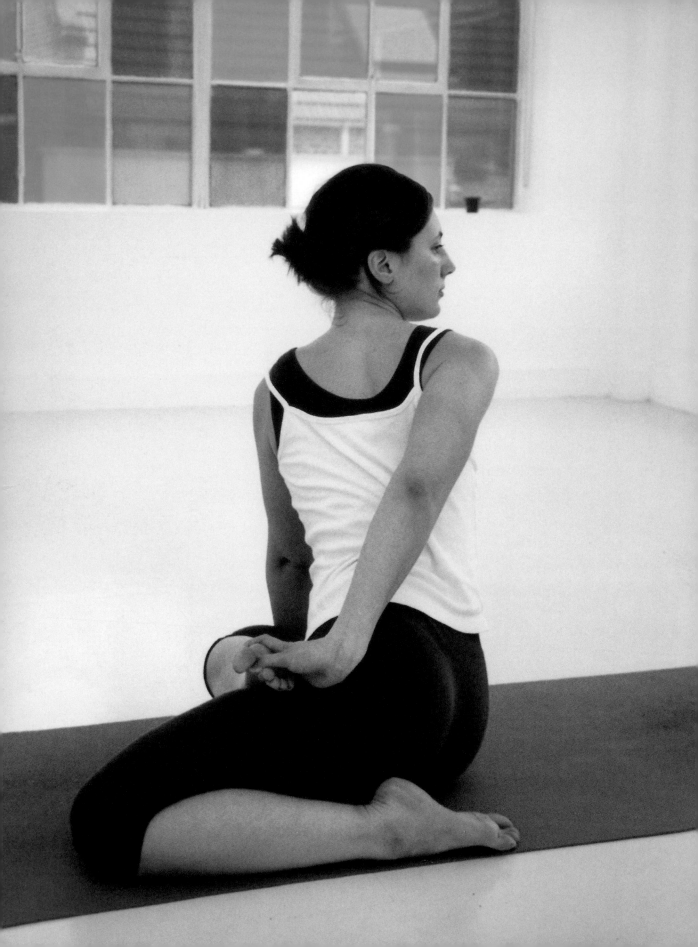

CHAPTER ONE
INTRODUCTION TO ASHTANGA

The Ashtanga Vinyasa Primary Series is a specific set of postures linked by the breath and always practiced in the same order. This yoga can be extremely challenging at first but with persistence you will experience deep changes on every level.

Physically the Primary Series realigns the skeletal system, develops strong muscles and flexible joints, increases lung capacity, improves the health and efficiency of the internal organs, and stimulates the immune system. By focusing on the combined rhythm of breath and movement you will improve the mind's ability to concentrate. Learning to face physical difficulty on a regular basis not only tempers the ego, but also provides a quiet sense of achievement and self-confidence that will filter through to other areas of your life.

Yoga is not a religion, but most people develop an increased sense of spiritual awareness and connection through their practice no matter what spiritual beliefs they hold, if any, when they first begin.

HISTORY OF YOGA

The practice of yoga probably began at least five thousand years ago in the Indus Valley in northern India. The people living on the banks of the Indus River were sophisticated, intelligent, and civilized. Their cities were well planned, with sanitation and plumbing rivaling those of the Romans. They appear to have been technologically skillful, and they traded with countries as far away as Mesopotamia. Images of Shiva in his role as Yogeshvara, the Lord of Yoga, found in the area, suggest that practices such as meditation were already known and taught.

Around 1500 B.C.E., the Indus Valley was invaded by Aryan tribes from the north, who imposed their own civilization and language on the existing culture. The Indian caste system may date from this time as part of an attempt to prevent a mixing of the cultures. There is no doubt, however, that the early spiritual traditions of the Indus Valley civilization were adopted by the Aryans. By the time written records appear in the form of the Hindu Vedas, the writing is in Sanskrit, the language of the Aryans.

The mixed Indian culture that emerged after the invasion was one in which both technological and philosophical knowledge were valued and sought after. "Forest Academies," or *ashrams*, were set up for the study of *Brahmavidya*—"the science and study of God."

Ashrams were attended by *rishis*, or "sages," who sought the underlying truth of human existence. The conclusions they reached are summarized by Aldous Huxley in his introduction to the *Bhagavad Gita*: "1. There is an infinite changeless reality beneath the world of change. 2. This same reality lies at the core of every human personality. 3. The purpose of life is to discover this reality experientially: that is, to realize God while here on earth" (Easwaran, 4).

Yoga is a complex spiritual tradition and science of life, based on the practices of these forest rishis. The practice of yoga has evolved over thousands of years. Many branches of yoga have developed to suit different human experiences and

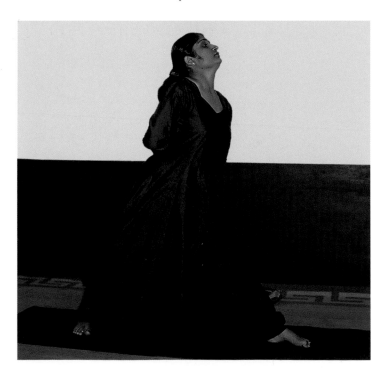

SHRUTI, SHARATH RANGASWAMIY'S WIFE, PRACTICING THE PRIMARY SERIES IN TRADITIONAL INDIAN ATTIRE IN 2001. WOMEN IN INDIA ARE STILL COVERING UP, WHEREAS WESTERN WOMEN WEAR SHORTS AND TIGHT TOPS TO ENABLE THEM TO DO VINYASAS EASILY.

temperaments, as is to be expected from such an ancient science.

Karma yoga is the yoga of action or work. Bhakti yoga is achieved by devotion to God. Jnâna yoga requires study and intellectual rigor to see beyond the illusions of life. Raja yoga is known as the way of meditation, but can include other forms of yoga. The path of Tantrism enlists the help of the feminine form of the divine, or Shakti, in the quest for liberation.

The form of yoga most familiar in the west is Hatha yoga. The word *hatha* represents the symbolic union between the sun (*ha*) and the moon (*tha*) and the balance between male and female, night and day, hard and soft. Hatha also means "forceful" and it relies on the practice of physical exercise to purify and strengthen the body to prepare it for liberation and enlightenment. Ashtanga Vinyasa yoga is a form of Hatha yoga.

The Sanskrit word *yoga* itself is derived from the root *yuj*, which means "to yoke or to unite." The many systems of yoga that have developed over the millennia are bound together by a common aim, which is to teach students a discipline that will eventually place them in direct contact with the divine.

Since yoga was first transmitted orally, it is impossible to know exactly when the practice of physical postures became linked with the spiritual quest of yoga. Hatha yoga

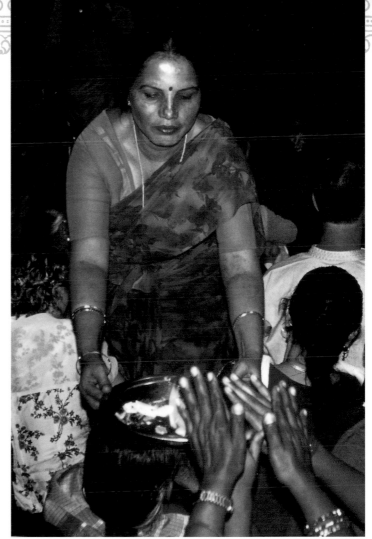

is probably an offshoot of Tantrism, which considers the body a temple of the divine and a valuable tool on the path to enlightenment. As such, it was originally based upon goddess worship and the awakening of Shakti energy (or *kundalini*) in the spine. One of the first Hatha yogis is said to have been a Punjabi sage called Goraksha, who lived approximately one thousand years ago. What is certain is that yoga is a living tradition, and the recent upsurge of interest in the West is contributing to and changing many aspects of the practice, making the benefits of yoga available to more people than ever before.

A PUJA CEREMONY TO MARK THE OPENING OF A TEMPLE BUILT BY GURUJI IN 2001 IN HONOR OF HIS BELOVED WIFE AMMA. HERE HIS DAUGHTER SARASWATI OFFERS A CEREMONIAL PLATE OF FIRE TO DEVOTEES.

THE STORY OF ASHTANGA

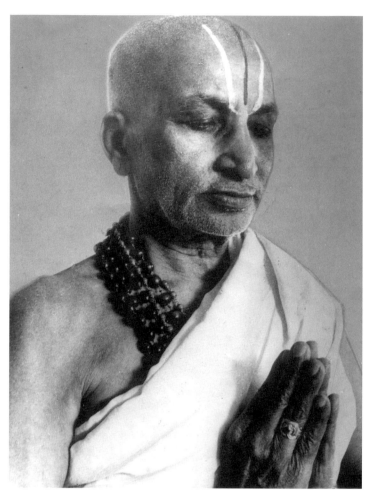

TIRUMALAI
KRISHNAMACHARYA, THE
"FATHER" OF ASHTANGA.

The great teacher Tirumalai Krishnamacharya was a pivotal force in the development of the various strands of yoga as we know it now, particularly Ashtanga Vinyasa Yoga. At the age of five, Krishnamacharya was initiated into Hatha yoga when his father began to teach him the great sage Patanjali's *sutras* (Vedic teachings). He also learned that his family was descended from a revered ninth-century yogi, Nathamuni. Many people who lead extraordinary lives experience one moment, an epiphany, that alters the course of their lives forever; for Krishnamacharya it was the experience of a vision at Nathamuni's shrine when he was 16. In the vision, he encountered his ancestor at the gates of the temple and was directed to a nearby mango grove. There he collapsed in an exhausted and altered state. When he arose he noticed three yogis before him with his ancestor seated in the middle. The adolescent boy then prostrated himself in honor of his ancestor and asked for instruction. For hours, Nathamuni sang verses to him from the *Yogarahasya*, which means "the essence of yoga" in Sanskrit. This text, allegedly lost for a thousand years, was the same text that Krishnamacharya memorized as it was passed to him in this mystical vision. Later he transcribed the ancient text and felt that he had become a divine instrument through which the teachings could manifest.

Krishnamacharya's thirst for study led him to seek out the master Sri Ramamohan Bramachari with whom he studied for seven years. During this time he memorized the *Yoga Sutra* of Patanjali and learned *asanas* (positions), *pranayama* (breathing), and the therapeutic qualities of yoga. He mastered three thousand asanas and feats of bodily control, such as stopping his pulse. As his reputation grew, he was invited to advise on cures for the maharajah's serious attacks of asthma. Through performing yoga work with the breath, the maharajah was cured. In gratitude he invited Krishnamacharya to teach at the Sanskrit College where the ruling family of Mysore had historically been patrons of the Indian arts and culture. The maharajah became his personal patron and supported the promotion of yoga throughout India. He later offered Krishnamacharya his own yoga *shala* (school) in the palace's gymnastics hall when it became clear that the yogi was so strict a disciplinarian that students at the Sanskrit College were complaining. This shala was to become the seat of Ashtanga Vinyasa Yoga.

When Guruji was a boy of 12, he attended one of Krishnamacharya's early demonstrations of yoga at the Jubilee Hall of Hassan, in southern India. Due to the influence of British colonial rule and its adverse effect on Indian traditions, Krishnamacharya had been earning little from his yogic abilities and had taken a job as a coffee plantation foreman. However, on his days off he continued his work of bringing yoga out of the shadows and showing the local populace some of the variations of yoga he had learned.

As one so young, Guruji had neither background nor understanding of the philosophy of yoga but, like many others who experience a calling, he was drawn toward his destiny. After seeing the demonstration, he was so impressed that he asked Krishnamacharya to teach him. In terms of the yogic spiritual belief system, he was fulfilling his *karma* (destiny). Those who now practice Ashtanga are aware of the belief that anyone who practices Ashtanga has done so before in a past life, as it is based on reincarnation. After being cross-examined and answering many questions from the gruff yogi, Guruji was requested to return the following day to start his studies. At the time no one in his own family was interested in yoga, as it was believed to be an esoteric system studied primarily by holy men who renounced family life. It was considered a reclusive path and one that did not nurture the family. As a Brahmin, Guruji was educated in Hindu rituals and also attended school. In order to learn yoga, he rose early and walked five kilometers to practice, then went to school afterward. He did this without his family's knowledge for two years, then went to study at the Sanskrit College in Mysore. By this time Krishnamacharya had been invited to teach at the college and so the two men continued what was to be a long-lasting relationship between master and student.

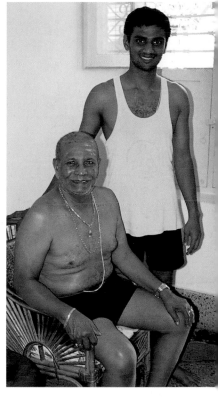

SRI K. PATTHABI JOIS (GURUJI), WITH HIS GRANDSON, SHARATH RANGASWAMY, THE WORLD'S MOST ADVANCED PRACTITIONER OF ASHTANGA.

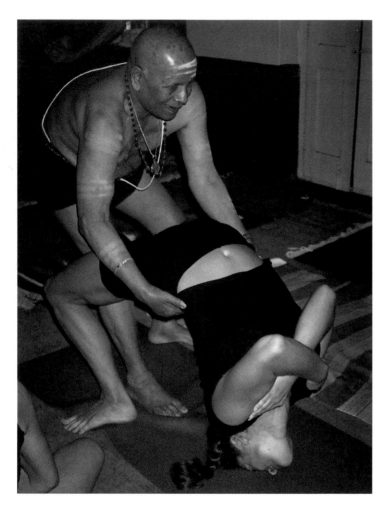

Krishnamacharya also used a stick to reprimand his students, yet Guruji himself never became a harsh teacher.

Guruji continues to teach this practice as it was taught in the 1930s when Ashtanga Vinyasa was first fully developed. He claims that the style originated with an ancient text called the *Yoga Kuruntha* that he himself never saw but that Krishnamacharya had read and later taught to him. Guruji also incorporates teachings from the *Hatha Yoga Pradipika*, the *Yoga Sutras* and the *Bhagavad Gita*, all famous yogic texts. Thus the style we now know as Ashtanga Vinyasa Yoga, or Mysore Style Ashtanga, is that which Krishnamacharya was teaching primarily to young boys in the 1930s. It reflects the athletic prowess and flexibility of the young male students and the fact that he had incorporated other disciplines such as gymnastics and Indian wrestling for the entertainment of the maharajah and other audiences.

A traditional Indian man, Krishnamacharya had little experience with women in anything other than the traditional roles of wife and mother; however, an interesting event led to women's inclusion in Ashtanga yoga training. A western woman was a friend of the maharajah's family in Mysore. Born Zhenia Labunskaia in pre-Soviet Latvia, she subsequently became known as Indra Devi. She too witnessed a demonstration by

GURUJI ASSISTING IN A DROPBACK WITH MICHAELA AT THE ASHTANGA YOGA RESEARCH INSTITUTE, MYSORE, INDIA.

When the yoga shala was granted by the maharajah of Mysore, Guruji became one of its most devoted students and advanced practitioners and as such was sent around the country to give demonstrations. Here Guruji also experienced the harsh side of his teacher. Krishnamacharya demanded absolute dedication and upheld it with punishments. If he was late by even one minute for a class, Guruji was made to stand out in the hot sun for half an hour.

Krishnamacharya at the palace and went to him for instruction. At first he refused and told her that he didn't teach foreigners or women. Undaunted, she persisted and persuaded the maharajah to speak to Krishnamacharya on her behalf. The reluctant teacher initially attempted to break her by giving her strict dietary rules and a difficult schedule. She met every challenge and during a year-long apprenticeship was an exemplary student. Eventually Krishnamacharya asked her to become a yoga teacher. He then spent days dictating yoga instruction, ayurvedic medicine, and pranayama. Devi became one of his best pupils as well as a good friend and paved the way for women to move forward in the yoga world. Her first best-selling book on Hatha yoga, published in 1953, is called *Forever Young, Forever Healthy*.[1] Devi went on to found the first school of yoga in Shanghai, China, and even opened up yoga in the Soviet Union (where it had been illegal) by convincing leaders that yoga was not a religion. In 1947 she moved to the U.S. and became known as the First Lady of Yoga, attracting students such as Gloria Swanson, Greta Garbo, Elizabeth Arden, and Marilyn Monroe.

Whereas Guruji adheres to the Ashtanga Vinyasa style of yoga as taught by Krishnamacharya, making only minor refinements, Indra Devi modified Ashtanga freely to create her own form of yoga. She used a more gentle approach to reflect the differences she experienced when Krishnamacharya in later years taught a highly individualized yoga in an attempt to simultaneously challenge and respect limitations. Her method does not incorporate *vinyasas* (linking movements), but it does consist of sequences of postures linked with the breath to create a journey from start to finish. She also introduced the idea of devotional invocation, calling her form of yoga *Sai yoga*. Indra Devi eventually moved to Buenos Aires, Argentina, where she opened six yoga schools. She taught well into her nineties, conducted world tours at an advanced age, and died in 2001 at the age of 103.

In contrast to other forms of yoga, Ashtanga yoga is often considered to be a hard and exacting path. Strength and stretch are used to move dynamically from one asana to the next, and most people develop muscles they never thought they had. Krishnamacharya was undoubtedly influenced by both Guruji and Indra Devi. As is often the case, the yoga teacher learns from the student as much as the student learns from the teacher, and it is a great spiritual wisdom that the best teachers meet those students who are meant to challenge them.

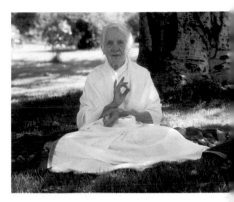

INDRA DEVI, THE FIRST FEMALE STUDENT OF ASHTANGA YOGA.

WHAT IS ASHTANGA VINYASA YOGA?

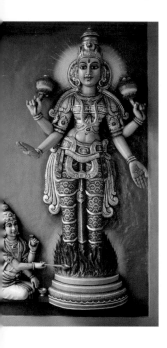

HINDU STATUE OF
A FEMALE DEITY.

The word *Ashtanga* means "eight limbs." The meaning of *Vinyasa* is "breath and movement combined for a specific purpose." In Ashtanga Vinyasa yoga we begin by combining breath and movement in a vigorous physical practice. In the words of Guruji, this form is "Ninety-nine percent practice and one percent theory." It is possible to achieve great benefits from this yoga purely through physical effort, but that does not mean that the theory is unimportant. The philosophy behind the practice can be inspiring in itself.

The eight limbs are the basis of many forms of yoga and were first documented more than two thousand years ago by a sage called Patanjali. No one is sure of Patanjali's true identity. Some say he was an incarnation of the divine serpent, Adishesha, who came to earth to instruct and enlighten human beings. He may have been a doctor, he certainly practiced yoga, and he was the first person to put into writing teachings that had until then been purely oral traditions passed from guru to student. Whatever his provenance, he was something of a renaissance man and wrote commentaries on grammar and medicine as well as on yoga.

Patanjali wrote four sets of aphorisms called the *Yoga Sutras*. In the Sutras he defined yoga in practical terms and explained how to use yoga practice to overcome the afflictions of the mind, reach a state of detachment, and ultimately attain full enlightenment.

The first two limbs of yoga are *Yama* and *Niyama*. They are suggestions for our behavior as humans in relationship to other living beings, our environment, and our selves. Although they have been compared to the Ten Commandments, rather than being divine law they are simply tools for improving our own lives and the lives of others. These two limbs are discussed in greater depth below.

The third limb of yoga is *Asana*, or the physical "postures." By practicing the asanas correctly we can minimize the effects of an unhealthy past and limit the impact of disease. Physical practice also stills the mind and can help to ease emotional difficulties.

The fourth limb of yoga is *Pranayama*, or "breath control." While we use *Ujjayi* pranayama throughout the Primary Series, advanced pranayama is not covered in this book, and in the Ashtanga system it is performed only by those practicing more advanced series. Nevertheless, using Ujjayi breath in the context of the Primary Series begins the process of stilling the mind, which will aid in the attainment of the final four limbs.

The first four limbs of Ashtanga yoga relate to the external environment and to the physical body. The remaining four limbs are internal and develop control of the mind, while relying on the physical and emotional processes begun with the practices of conscious living, care of the body, and attention to the breath.

The fifth limb of yoga is *Pratayahara*, which literally means "control of the senses." When we start to practice yoga, we may find it difficult to achieve control, even of the body. Through constant and regular practice the will becomes stronger and is able to release the "chattering in the brain" that keeps us from addressing challenging situations and obscures our clarity of purpose.

The sixth limb, *Dharana*, or "concentration," progresses naturally from the ability to control the senses. The ability to focus on one specific goal and direct the mind at will leads us to a state of *Dhyana*, or "meditation," the seventh limb of yoga. In a state of meditation we direct our mind to the exclusion of other thoughts.

The final and eighth limb of yoga and the ultimate goal of our practice is *Samadhi*, or "bliss." In Samadhi the effort that was required of us for practicing the preceding seven limbs disappears as we find that the barriers that have been erected between our conscious mind and that of the divine are melting effortlessly and wordlessly away.

YAMA & NIYAMA

The first of the eight limbs of yoga, *Yama*, means "self-restraint" and consists of instructions for successful interaction with our environment. The second limb, Niyama, is intended to develop a similar attitude toward our selves. Although the *Yoga Sutras* were written in a culture far removed from our own, the teachings of the Yamas and Niyamas are compatible with modern western thought and are useful for creating a fulfilling existence at a time where moral guidelines may be few and far between.

Moral codes are vital not only to the practice of yoga. The freedoms of thought and action that we take for granted in democratic society, flawed though they may be, spring from the same sense of right over might and self-respect that are the essence of the Yamas and Niyamas. These are universal principles to be followed by all regardless of age, class, or gender. Following these instructions will help you to achieve the correct state of mind to reach Samadhi. Their only purpose is to help you to evolve to the best of your ability.

YAMA

To practice Yama is to practice self-restraint in dealing with the outside world. The five principles of Yama are *Ahimsa*, *Satya*, *Ashteya*, *Brahmacharya*, and *Aparigraha*. Practicing *Ahimsa* means "striving not to harm any living thing," whether human or animal, in thought, word, or deed. For most

Two things fill the mind with ever new and increasing wonder and awe... the starry heaven above me, and the moral law within me.
EMMANUEL KANT

people, eating wholesome vegetarian food, noticing and avoiding spiteful thoughts and gossip, and addressing self-destructive tendencies such as eating disorders are steps in the right direction. When we abandon our own aggression we make it possible for others to relax in our presence and peaceful relationships can be established.

Satya, "truthfulness," is a powerful tool. If we say what we mean and mean what we say, we can harness the power to create our own reality and change our lives for the better. Being truthful in our yoga practice may mean going the extra bit farther in a posture rather than being lazy and only going through the motions—or it might mean accepting the need to move carefully rather than risk injury.

Ashteya, "not stealing," means not stealing the possessions of others, not being envious, and not using false pretenses to gain either tangibles or intangibles such as property, love, time, or energy from others. If you take what belongs to others you are not only doing wrong to them, but you will never be wholly trusted. By stealing you are assuming that abundance will not come to you naturally. Only when you stop coveting others' possessions and achievements can you appreciate what you already have and get what you really need.

Brahmacharya is commonly translated as "chastity." The literal meaning of the word is "student of God." Traditionally yoga

has been practiced by married people, and Guruji has outlined specific rules regarding appropriate times for sex. In the *Yoga Mala*, he also recommends avoiding those people who distract you from your path or drag you down emotionally. Historically some of the information about Brahmacharya was written by and for men and advised against ejaculation.

Sexual abstinence may bring freedom to some, but for many it can be as distracting as sexual obsession. T.K.V. Desikachar, son of Krishnamacharya, has written a very simple commentary on the *Sutras* in which he suggests that Brahmacharya simply means "moderation." B.K.S. Iyengar, in *Light on the Yoga Sutras of Patanjali*, points out that sexual energy is sacred and that only when pleasure is the sole motivation for sex is Brahmacharya violated. When a relationship is based on love, cooperation, and mutual support, sex can only enhance the experience. Practicing Brahmacharya will free the mind to focus on yoga and fill the body with energy.

Aparigraha, "freedom from greed," helps to liberate the mind. Our attachment to physical possessions is one of the greatest distractions we can experience as human beings. We spend much of our lives surrounding ourselves with things, protecting them, and planning new acquisitions. If we can avoid these tendencies, we will become free to contemplate the real meaning of our lives.

NIYAMA

Niyama relates to the development and evolution of the self. The five Niyamas are *Saucha*, *Santosha*, *Tapas*, *Svadhyaya*, and *Ishvara pranidhana*.

The meaning of *Saucha* is "cleanliness." Although the body is temporary, it houses the soul, which is eternal. As the home of the soul, the body is a temple. The process of cleaning the body, not only with soap and water, but also through the use of asanas and pranayama, is a discipline that encourages the pursuit of spiritual knowledge. A clean diet also helps. When first beginning Ashtanga yoga, students who habitually eat meat or fish, smoke tobacco, or take drugs express a most unpleasant odor. After only a few months of healthy living and regular practice, their sweat becomes sweet and odor free. When we are clean we feel awake, joyful, and ready to look within.

Santosha, "contentment," arises when we have cleansed our bodies and worked hard at the practice. The pure happiness of Santosha is not dependent on possessions or on the opinion of other people. It comes from the understanding that we are following a valid path that will lead us to self-realization.

Tapas, or "self-discipline," drives the whole process of yoga forward. Being motivated to do our practice allows body, mind, and spirit to be perfected, but for the best results we need to be honest with ourselves. Self-discipline will allow the practice to unfold as it should.

Svadhyaya means "study which leads to knowledge of the self." In Ashtanga Vinyasa yoga we learn most of our lessons on the mat. We learn about courage, commitment, surrender, and faith. The yoga practice highlights our strengths and weaknesses. We challenge ourselves daily and reaffirm our intentions.

Ishvara pranidhana, the final Niyama, means "faith." In accepting our limitations and surrendering our will to a higher power, we can liberate the soul from the restraints of the conscious mind and allow ourselves to experience the perfection of Samadhi.

At first the task of following the Yamas and Niyamas can seem daunting, but Guruji has suggested that by practicing the physical form of Astanga Vinyasa yoga, the student will gain clarity of thought, strength of mind, and motivation to change. Observing the Yamas and Niyamas will then come naturally, whether the student is aware of this development or not.

Renounce and enjoy!

GANDHI

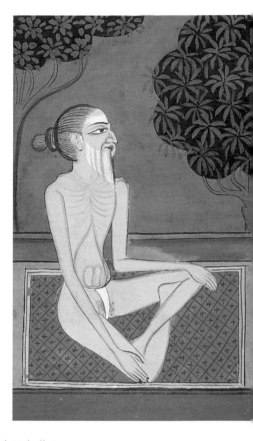

ILLUSTRATED EXAMPLE OF YOGA BEING PRACTICED IN ANCIENT INDIA.

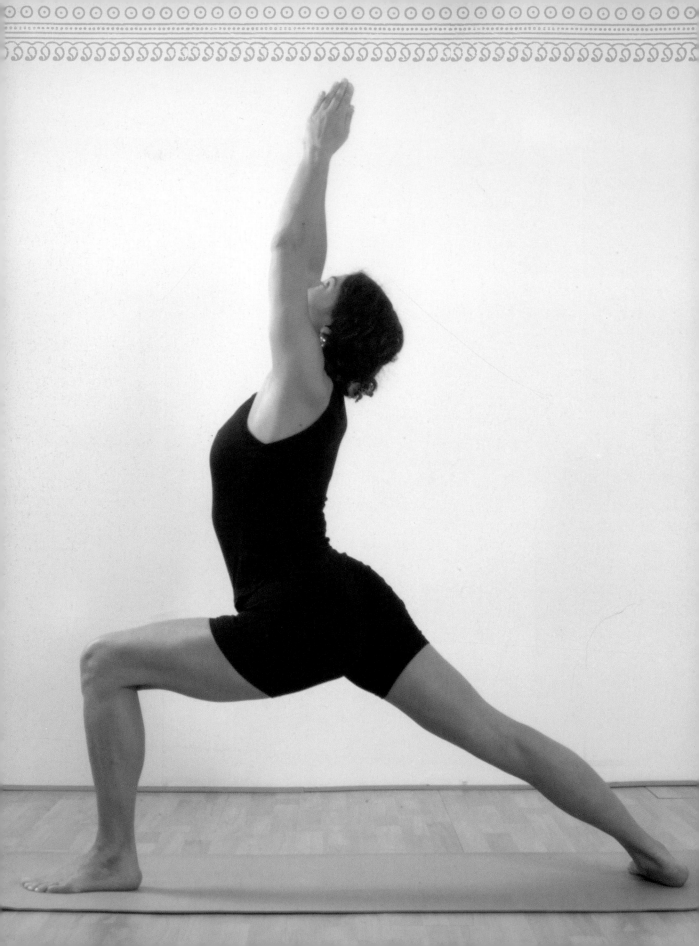

CHAPTER TWO

THE PRIMARY SERIES

Below is the traditional mantra that is chanted at the beginning of Ashtanga yoga practice.
It is always recited in Sanskrit. However, you may wish to choose your own prayer or affirmation.

Om

Vande Gurunam Charanaravinde

Sandarshita svatma sukava bodhe

Nishreyase Jangalikayamane

Samsara halahala mohashantiyai

Abahu Purushakaram

Shankhachakrasi dharinam

Sahasra shirasam shvetam

Pranamami Patanjalim

Om

Om

I pray at the lotus feet of the supreme guru

Who illuminates the path to enlightenment

And like a doctor of the jungle

Removes the poison of conditioned existence.

To the sage Patanjali, an incarnation of

White Adishesha with a thousand radiant

heads in the form of the divine serpent,

Ananta, Human below the shoulders,

Holding a sword of discrimination, a fiery

wheel meaning infinite time

And a conch representing divine sound

I surrender

Om

PREPARATIONS FOR PRACTICE

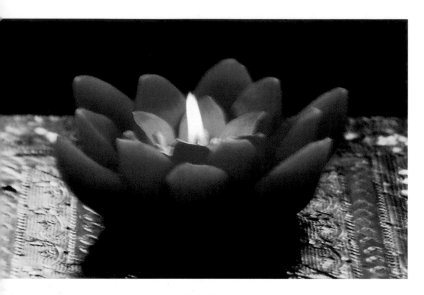

LOTUS FLOWER CANDLE
USED FOR MEDITATION.
THE LOTUS FLOWER
IS A TRADITIONAL
YOGA SYMBOL.

The best time to practice yoga is before sunrise after emptying the bowels and bathing. Whenever you practice you should do so on an empty stomach (at least three or four hours after eating) and you should refrain from drinking during the practice. Do remember to drink plenty of water during the day to replace fluids lost while sweating. Cleanliness is important not only because it minimizes body odor, but also because warm water can ease sore muscles and prepare the skin to sweat efficiently.

Ancient yoga texts suggest building a yoga hut with a level mud floor covered in hides and safe from wild animals in a forest far from the distractions of society. Today all you need is an area large enough for your mat with enough room to stretch your arms to the sides and above your head. It is a good idea to dedicate a particular space to your yoga. You can also use flowers, candles, and devotional art to set the mood. Some people like to play music, but for beginners it is important to focus on the sound of the breath until it becomes easy and natural.

The best mats to use for Ashtanga Vinyasa yoga are sticky mats, which are widely available, and many people use a woven cotton mat on top to absorb perspiration. Wear comfortable clothes that allow for ease of motion and tie your hair back if it is long.

Begin your practice by standing up straight at the front of the mat with your back straight, your neck in line with your spine, your feet together, and your arms comfortably at your sides. This position is called Samasthitih, or Neutral Pose. Clear your mind, listen to your breath, and prepare to focus fully on the exercises. Let go of any negative emotions and be willing to move forward. Bring your hands into prayer position, close your eyes, and prepare your thoughts.

It is usual to begin a yoga practice with a mantra or prayer. The traditional Ashtanga yoga mantra, as taught by Guruji in Mysore and shown on page 21, can be used, or you may prefer to choose a simple prayer or affirmation of your own.

Open your eyes when you have finished, look at your nose, and begin your breathing and bandhas.

DANCING TO THE MUSIC OF THE BREATH

Breathing is our most basic act as living human beings. We begin our lives on earth with our first breath and exit on our last. The breath is an essential connection to the world and expresses and informs our every mood and emotion. When we are excited or scared, breathing becomes shallow and quick; deep breathing will calm the mind and soothe the body. We can allow the breath to master us, or we can use breathing techniques to control our responses to anything from activities in the outside world to unwanted thoughts.

When practicing the postures of the Ashtanga Vinyasa sequence, the breath is used consciously to link the movements and measure time in the postures. The sound of the breath is continuous and rhythmic, an unbroken chain of inhalation and exhalation. When you move you will be dancing to the music of the breath without pause from the beginning to the end of your practice.

The process of linking breath and movement is called *Vinyasa*. Someone who has been practicing for some time will be adept at flowing through the Primary Series using the correct Vinyasa as is described in the following chapter. In other words, they will not need to take extra breaths while going into and coming out of the postures.

However, even the most proficient student needs to take extra breaths sometimes when working into difficult or new positions.

It is possible to take extra breaths without interrupting the flow of the practice if the basic principles of breath and movement are observed. As a rule, all lifts, extensions, opening or upward movements, and backbends are performed on an inhalation. All downward, backward, folding, twisting, or contracting movements are performed on an exhalation. For example, you inhale to extend the spine, and exhale to fold forward. The key to taking extra breaths during the practice is to take them consciously, match them to an appropriate movement, and keep them the same length as the rest of the breathing. It is much better to pause for extra breaths than to hold the breath or rush into the posture incorrectly.

Chapter Two breaks down the yoga practice breath by breath, as it is usually taught. For less advanced students extra breaths are suggested in parenthesis.

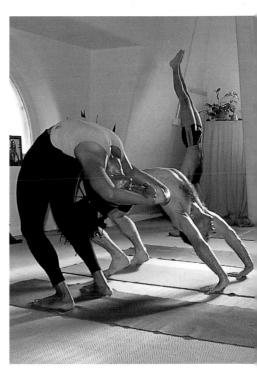

THROUGH THE BREATH, STUDENTS MOVE AT THEIR OWN PACE THROUGH MORNING PRACTICE.

BREATHING

It is worth taking time at the beginning to get the breathing right. The breath performs many functions and is essential to the effectiveness of the yoga practice.

Throughout the practice a particular breathing style called *Ujjayi breathing* is used. *Ujjayi* means "victorious," and this breath is designed to help you overcome both physical and emotional obstacles.

Ujjayi breath has a distinctive sibilant sound made by contracting the muscles at the back of the throat. The first stage in learning the breath is to breathe through your nose and to count, if necessary, so that the inhalation and the exhalation are the same length with no pauses between breaths. When we breathe normally the exhalation tends to be longer, so you will need to speed up the exhalation and slow the inhalation. This should encourage you to breathe more deeply.

Next clear your throat. The same muscles you use to clear your throat are the muscles that you will contract slightly in Ujjayi breathing. The only difference is that you will only contract them halfway.

Practice until your breath is smooth but easily audible on both inhalation and exhalation. You may need to clear your throat a few times to remind you of the muscles used.

Beginners often find that they make strange noises or cannot make any noise at all, but with practice this breath can be mastered by anyone.

There are several reasons for contracting the throat in this way. It helps to relieve pressure in the nasal passages, preventing them from blocking up and allowing a faster flow of air to the lungs. This is particularly important for beginners who may get out of breath during the Sun Salutations. Keeping pressure in the throat also allows breath to be drawn in evenly through both nostrils. In addition to this the air is heated slightly on the inhalation, helping to increase overall body temperature which will improve flexibility. Being able to hear the breath emphasizes its importance while moving through the postures; the sound also serves as a tool for focusing the mind.

In general each of the postures is held for five breaths. When a particular posture is required for its therapeutic benefits, it may be held for up to 25 breaths.

BANDHA

Bandha means "lock" or "seal." In this context it is a muscular contraction at specific points in the body throughout the practice. In the primary series two bandhas are used, Mula Bandha and Uddiyana Bandha.

Mula Bandha is the "root lock" and is achieved by contracting the anal sphincter muscles. In women it can also be helpful

BENEFITS: In addition to its general benefits performing Ujjayi breathing while seated in a comfortable position is often helpful in relieving menstrual cramps.

FULL LOTUS POSITION IS HELD FOR 25 BREATHS AT THE END OF THE PRIMARY SERIES.

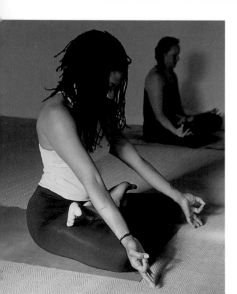

to contract the cervix. Guruji says that when you can control the anus, you can control your mind, and Mula Bandha does require a great deal of concentration. Practice Mula Bandha by exhaling completely, squeeze in the sphincter muscles, and while you inhale, continue to draw up and in through the anus. Developing Mula Bandha will help tone the pelvic floor and vagina, improve bladder control, and support the uterus and lower digestive organs. Mula Bandha is emphasized while jumping, since the upward direction of energy will help you "fly." Contracting this bandha during challenging postures will also help relax the rest of the body and relieve pain.

Uddiyana Bandha means "upward flying seal." It is an inward and upward contraction of the lower abdomen so that it remains lightly drawn in and still throughout the breath. The area above the navel should continue to move freely with the breath. When the abdominal muscles are contracted in this way they support and protect the lower back. By drawing in the lower abdomen on the inhalation the lungs are forced to expand out toward the ribs rather than down into the abdomen, which will help increase lung capacity and cardiovascular fitness. The use of Uddiyana Bandha also provides resistance to the diaphragm, which then massages the internal organs, allowing fresh blood to circulate and improving the efficiency of the spleen, liver, and digestive system.

DRISHTI

Drishti means "gaze point." Drishti is used to encourage correct form in each posture and to help with mental focus. It is important to remember to practice the drishti.

Nasagrai (**nose**): This drishti is used while standing in Neutral Pose, while moving into Upward Dog to prevent overextension of the neck, and in several other postures as a means to avoid distraction.

Anjusta ma dyai (**thumbs**): Used when extending the arms in order to emphasize the upward motion of the body or, as in the case of Trikonasana (Triangle pose), to encourage the chest to open.

Broomadhya (**Third Eye**): This gaze also encourages the upward and opening motion of the body and lengthening of the spine.

Nabi chakra (**navel**): In Downward Dog, we look at the navel by tucking the chin into the collarbone to still the mind.

Urdhva (**upward**): This is an opening drishti.

Hastagrai (**hand**): This gaze point is used to encourage correct alignment in extended postures.

Padhayoragrai (**toes**): In forward bends, it is important to look at your toes so that your spine will lengthen naturally.

Parsva (**to the side**): This focus is used during both balancing and twisting postures.

PRACTICING NASAGRAI (GAZING AT THE NOSE) WHILE HOLDING BOUND LOTUS.

BENEFITS: Women suffering from a prolapsed uterus will find the bandhas helpful.

THE SUN SALUTATIONS

Once you have mastered the breath and come to understand bandha and drishti, you should proceed to the Sun Salutations. The Sun Salutations are originally devotional in nature, but they also have the effect of warming up the body by taking it breath by breath through a full range of motion, pausing only in Downward Dog to begin easing the muscles in the back and legs. You will develop strength, flexibility, stamina, and breath control. One of the main premises of this practice is that in order to work safely to your edge, you must be hot, preferably sweating. The Sun Salutations will heat you up.

Sun Salute A has nine Vinyasas, or simple moves to the breath, that kick-start the process of preparing body, mind, and spirit for what is to come by stretching and strengthening the arms and legs and by working the spine forward and backward to invigorate the nervous system. Sun Salute B flows in the same way but with 17 Vinyasas, including movements that will begin to open the hips and shoulders and strengthen the spine.

SURYA NAMASKARA A
SUN SALUTE A

BENEFITS: This sequence heats the body, stretches and strengthens the arms, legs, hands, feet, wrists, and ankles, and assists in the healthy development of the chest. Upward Dog stretches the spine, chest, and quadriceps and Downward Dog stretches the calves and opens the shoulders. These movements, combined with breathing and bandha, tone the reproductive system and can ease the symptoms of menopause.

Jumping strengthens the knee joints, improves coordination and stamina, and relieves depression and lethargy. It will also help increase bone density and prevent osteoporosis.

> **TIP:** If you are unable to jump forward or backward into postures, begin by stepping or walking into them one foot at a time. Take extra breaths where necessary (never hold the breath). Occasionally practice jumping, remembering to activate the bandhas, and build up your strength in your own time.

Begin by standing in Neutral Pose at the front of your mat.

❶ **INHALE:** Reach up with straight arms, bringing your palms together. Look up at your thumbs.

❷ **EXHALE:** Fold forward from your hips, bring your hands to the floor shoulder distance apart, and tuck in your head. Look at your nose.

> **TIP:** If you can't get your hands to the floor, bend your knees to bring them flat. This will help release the muscles of your lower back.

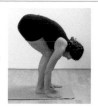

❸ **INHALE:** Lift your head to open your chest and extend your spine. Look up.

> **CONTRAINDICATIONS:** DO NOT JUMP WHEN PREGNANT OR WHEN SUFFERING FROM KNEE OR BACK INJURIES.

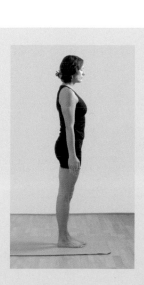

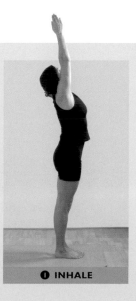

❶ INHALE

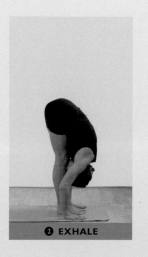

❷ EXHALE

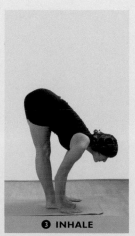

❸ INHALE

④ EXHALE: Jump back, feet hip distance apart, to a push-up position. Bend your elbows, keeping your upper arms parallel to the floor and back straight. Bring your chin an inch from the floor, keeping your chest, pelvis, and knees off the floor. This is Chatturanga Dandasana or All Fours Staff position. Look at your nose.

MODIFICATION

Many women do not have the upper body strength necessary to lower into All Fours Staff position without collapsing in the pelvis. This should be avoided as it can cause pain in the lower back. Instead, bend your knees and bring them to the floor in a "ladies' push-up" position, before attempting to lower your chin and chest to strengthen your arms.

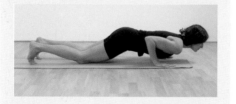

⑤ INHALE: Push your chest forward, straighten your arms, and roll over your toes into Upward Dog. Make sure that your knees and hips are off the floor. Look at your nose.

> **TIP:** Rolling over your toes will happen naturally if you keep your feet where they are and come into Upward Dog by pressing your chest forward.

⑥ EXHALE: Push your buttocks up and roll over your toes into Downward Dog. Look toward your navel. **Hold Downward Dog for 5 breaths**.

> **TIP:** In Downward Dog hands are shoulder distance apart, feet are hip distance apart and parallel. Back, arms, and legs are straight and shoulders and back are broad. To look toward your navel, tuck your chin into your collarbone. Focus on Uddiyana Bandha and correct breathing. On the fifth exhale prepare to spring by activating Mula Bandha and bending your knees slightly.

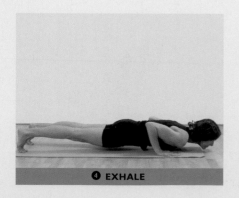

④ EXHALE

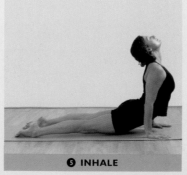

⑤ INHALE

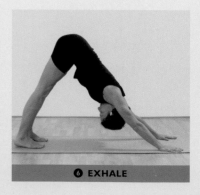

⑥ EXHALE

❼ INHALE: Jump forward, landing with feet together between your hands, then straighten your legs. Look up.

❽ EXHALE: Fold in toward your legs. Look at your nose.

> MODIFICATION
> Walk your feet forward if jumping is not possible.

❾ INHALE: Come all the way up, bringing your arms over your head, palms together. Look up at your thumbs.

EXHALE: Bring your arms down to your sides to return to Neutral Pose. Look at your nose.

Repeat Sun Salute A at least 5 times without pausing. Make sure you have mastered it before moving on.

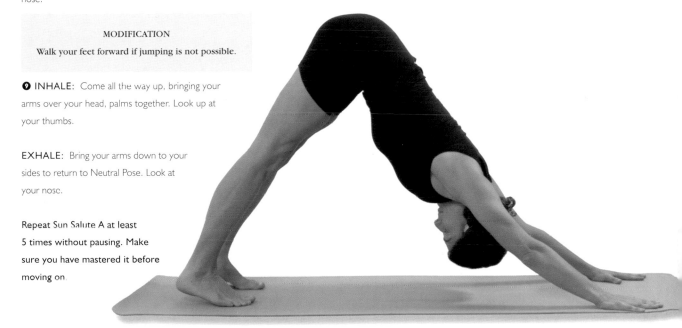

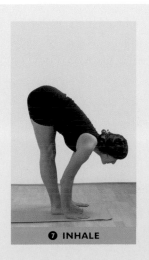

❼ INHALE

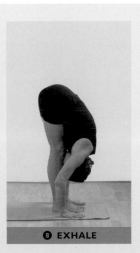

❽ EXHALE

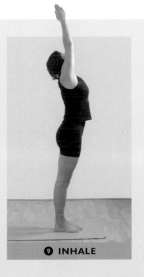

❾ INHALE

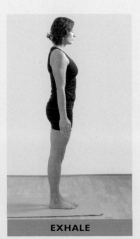

EXHALE

SURYA NAMASKARA B
SUN SALUTE B

BENEFITS: Sun Salute B promotes increased strength in the lower back, flexibility in the hips, and greater powers of endurance.

> **CONTRAINDICATIONS**: DO NOT JUMP WHEN PREGNANT OR WHEN SUFFERING FROM KNEE OR BACK INJURIES.

❶ INHALE: From Neutral Pose, bend your knees deeply, keeping your heels down, reach up with straight arms, and bring your palms together. Look up at your thumbs.

❷ EXHALE: Bring your hands to the floor, shoulder distance apart. Straighten your legs and tuck in your head. Look at your nose.

❸ INHALE: Lift your head to open your chest and extend your spine. Look up.

❹ EXHALE: Jump back, feet hip distance apart, to a push-up position. Bend your elbows and bring your chin an inch from the floor, keeping your chest, pelvis, and knees off the floor. Look at your nose.

❺ INHALE: Push your chest forward, straighten your arms, and roll over your toes into Upward Dog. Look at your nose.

❻ EXHALE: Push your buttocks up and roll over your toes into Downward Dog. Before the end of the exhalation, turn the heel of your left foot toward the ball of your right foot and step your right foot between your hands. Keep your heels in line. Your right leg should be bent at a 90-degree angle so your knee is directly above your ankle. Your left leg is straight.

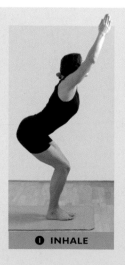

❶ INHALE

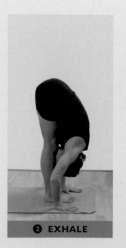

❷ EXHALE

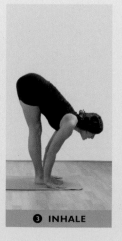

❸ INHALE

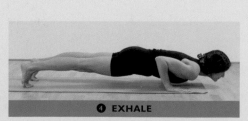

❹ EXHALE

TIPS: If you cannot step between your hands, try stepping forward before turning in your back foot. If this does not work, you can lower your back knee to the floor to step forward, then turn that heel in and lift and straighten the leg into position. Eventually you will develop the muscles and flexibility to step forward easily.

It is important to pay attention to both knees when working quickly into this Warrior position. To avoid twisting your knee, make sure that your back foot points slightly forward and remains on the floor while you arekeeping your back leg straight.Your front knee should remain vertically over your ankle.

❼ INHALE: Reach up, bringing your palms together. Arms and spine are vertical, hips and shoulders face evenly forward. Look up at your thumbs.

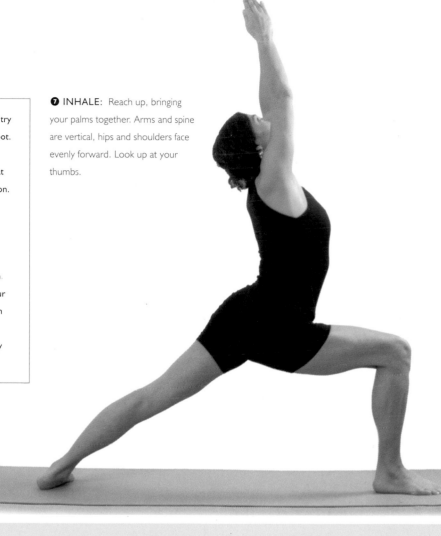

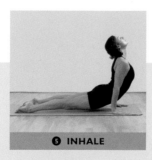

❺ INHALE

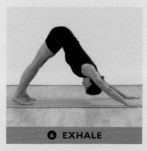

❻ EXHALE

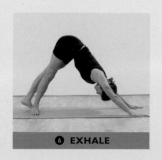

❻ EXHALE

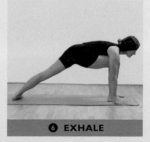

❻ EXHALE

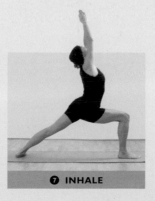

❼ INHALE

❽ EXHALE: Return your hands to the floor on either side of your right foot. Step back to a push-up position. Bend your elbows to keep your upper arms parallel to the floor and your back straight. Look at your nose.

❾ INHALE: Push your chest forward, straighten your arms, and roll over your toes into Upward Dog. Look at your nose.

❿ EXHALE: Push your buttocks up and roll over your toes into Downward Dog. Before the end of the exhalation, turn the heel of your right foot toward the ball of your left foot and step your left foot between your hands. Keep your heels in line. Your left leg should be bent at a 90-degree angle so your knee is directly above your ankle. Your right leg is straight.

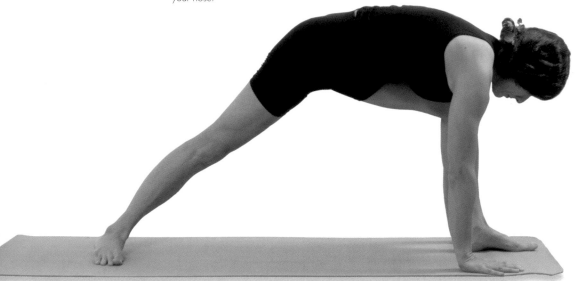

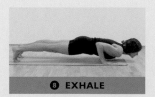
❽ EXHALE

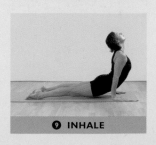
❾ INHALE

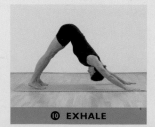
❿ EXHALE

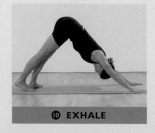
❿ EXHALE

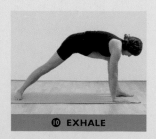
❿ EXHALE

⓫ INHALE: Reach up, bringing your palms together. Arms and spine are vertical, hips and shoulders face evenly forward. Look up at your thumbs.

⓬ EXHALE: Hands return to the floor on either side of your left foot. Step back to a push-up position. Bend your elbows to keep your upper arms parallel to the floor and your back straight. Look at your nose.

⓭ INHALE: Push your chest forward, straighten your arms, and roll over your toes into Upward Dog. Look at your nose.

⓮ EXHALE: Push your buttocks up and roll over your toes into Downward Dog. Look toward your navel. **Hold Downward Dog for 5 breaths as with Sun Salute A.**

⓯ INHALE: Jump forward, landing with feet together between your hands, and straighten your legs. Look up.

⓰ EXHALE: Fold in toward your legs. Look at your nose.

⓱ INHALE: Bend your knees deeply, keeping your heels down. With your knees bent, come all the way up, bringing your arms over your head, palms together. Look up at your thumbs.

⓲ EXHALE: Straighten your legs and bring your arms down to your sides to return to Neutral Pose. Look at your nose.

Repeat 5 times.

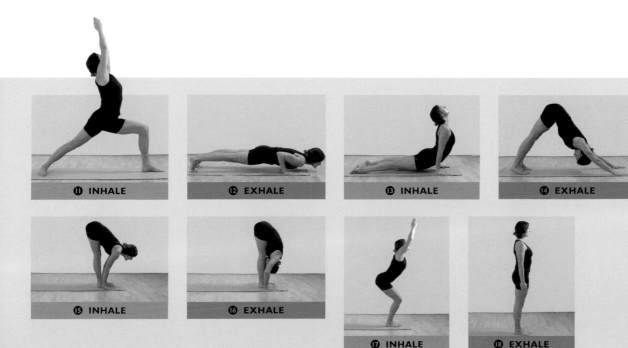

⓫ INHALE ⓬ EXHALE ⓭ INHALE ⓮ EXHALE

⓯ INHALE ⓰ EXHALE ⓱ INHALE ⓲ EXHALE

THE STANDING POSTURES

These postures begin the work of the practice. They help develop awareness of alignment. They stretch, strengthen, and relieve tension in the entire body. The waist is toned, and the internal organs are stimulated and regulated.

All of the asanas in Ashtanga Vinyasa yoga are done in sequential order, always working the right side first. Postures should not be missed out or taken out of context, as each one will prepare the body to safely attempt those that follow.

If you have a stiff body, it may be beneficial to work on only the Sun Salutations and Standing Postures to begin with, possibly repeating the sequence if a longer session is desired, in order to build a solid basis for the practice of the Primary Series which consists of the Sitting Postures.

PADANGUSTHASANA
BOUND TOE FORWARD BEND

❶ INHALE: From Neutral Pose, jump your feet hip distance apart, keeping your feet parallel. Place your hands on your waist, opening your chest.

> **TIP:** Every time you bring your hands to your waist, squeeze your fingers into your lower abdomen to assist you in drawing in and up on Uddiyana Bandha. When moving into forward bends, set Uddiyana Bandha on the inhale as preparation for coming forward and to protect your lower back, then draw up on Mula Bandha as you exhale forward and down.

❷ EXHALE: Fold forward and grasp your big toes with the first two fingers and thumb of each hand. Look at your nose.

> **MODIFICATION**
> In any forward bends where it is not possible to reach your toes, it is better to bend your knees to work into the posture, thereby helping to release the muscles of your lower back and hips, before attempting to straighten your legs.

❸ INHALE: Lift your head, shoulders, and chest. Extend through your spine. Look up

❹ EXHALE: Fold in toward your legs, drawing your head down and bringing your belly to your thighs, chest to your knees. Look at your nose. **Hold for 5 breaths.**

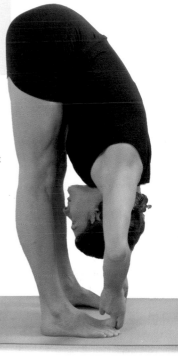

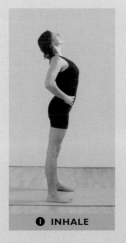
❶ INHALE

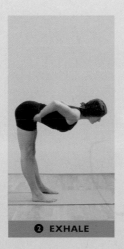
❷ EXHALE

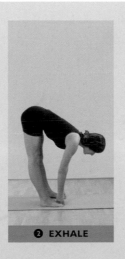
❷ EXHALE

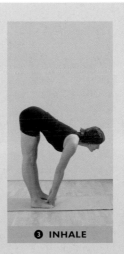
❸ INHALE

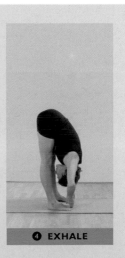
❹ EXHALE

PADAHASTASANA
HAND-TO-FOOT FORWARD BEND

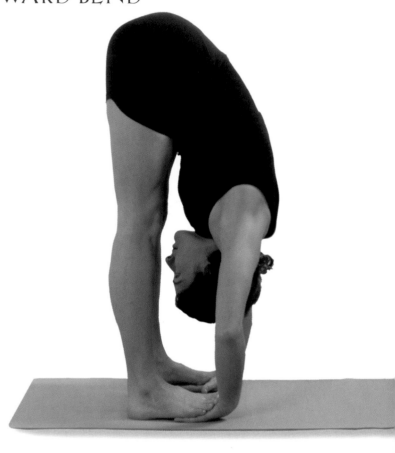

BENEFITS: This is particularly good during menstruation or when suffering from a prolapse of the uterus.

❶ INHALE: From Padangusthasana, straighten your arms, keeping the toe grip. Look up.

❷ EXHALE: Bring your hands all the way under the front of your feet and press down with your toes.

> TIP: Bend your knees and make sure your toes come all the way to your wrists rather than just standing on your fingers as this is a wrist stretch.

❸ INHALE: Lift your head, shoulders, and chest. Extend through your spine. Look up.

❹ EXHALE: Fold in toward your legs, drawing your head down and bringing your belly to your thighs, chest to your knees. Look at your nose. **Hold for 5 breaths.**

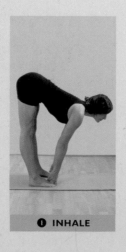
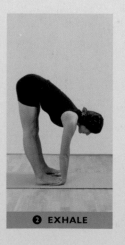
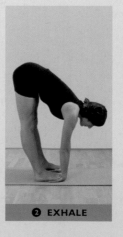
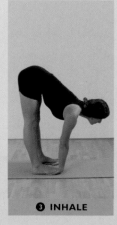
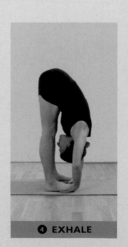

❶ INHALE   ❷ EXHALE   ❷ EXHALE   ❸ INHALE   ❹ EXHALE

5 INHALE: Look up.

6 EXHALE: Bring your hands to your waist. Look at your nose.

7 INHALE: Come all the way up.

8 EXHALE: Jump back to the Neutral Pose, landing with your feet together.

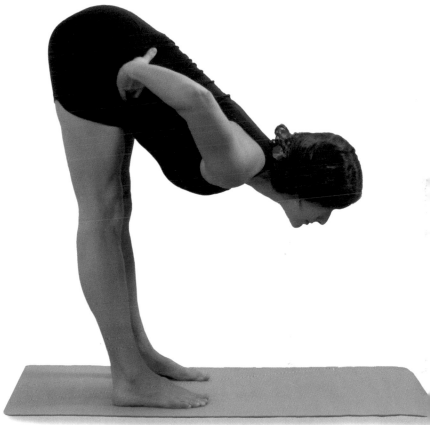

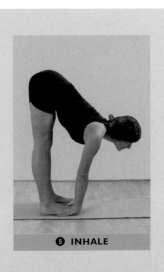
5 INHALE

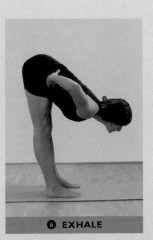
6 EXHALE

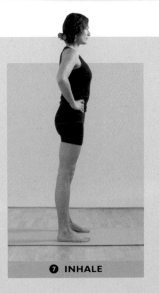
7 INHALE

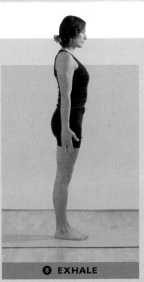
8 EXHALE

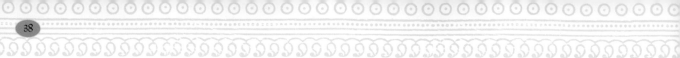

UTTHITA TRIKONASANA
EXTENDED TRIANGLE

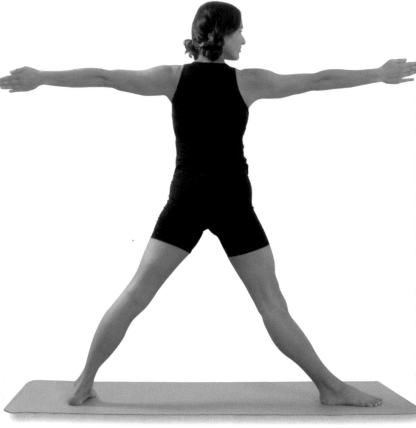

BENEFITS: Reaching to the side teaches alignment and a sense of direction. The reproductive and digestive systems are toned.

MODIFICATION
If pregnant, only go as far as is comfortable and work on lengthening from pubic bone to sternum.

❶ INHALE: From Neutral Pose, jump 90 degrees to the right, arms straight out to the sides, landing with your feet apart, parallel under your elbows. Turn your head to the right and and your right foot out 90 degrees, keeping your heels lined up.

❷ EXHALE: Fold to the right and grasp your right big toe with the first two fingers and thumb of your right hand. Watch where you are going.

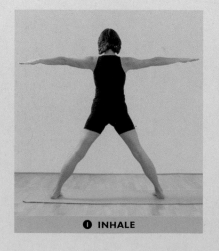

❶ INHALE

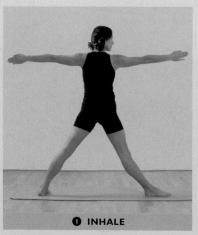

❶ INHALE

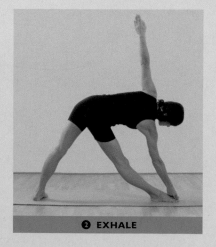

❷ EXHALE

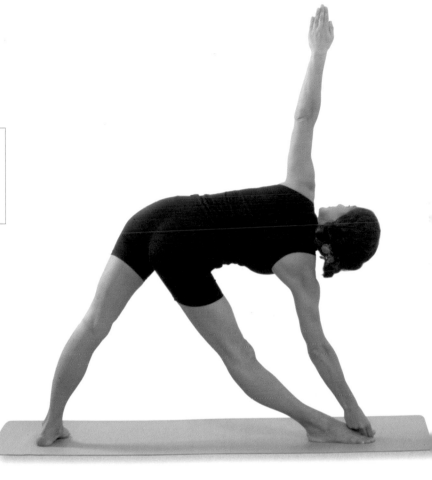

> **TIP:** If you are not flexible enough to reach your toe with your front leg straight, then bend your knee, work on your alignment, and finally work on straightening your leg while holding your toe.

❸ INHALE: Reach up with your left arm. Look at your left thumb.

❹ EXHALE: Work on bringing your left hip back in line with your right hip, and keeping your arms, chest and shoulders vertically in line. Hold the posture for 5 breaths.

❺ INHALE: Come up. Keep your arms extended. Turn your right foot to be parallel with your left, then turn your left foot out 90 degrees.

❻ EXHALE: Repeat the posture on the left side.

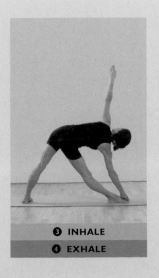
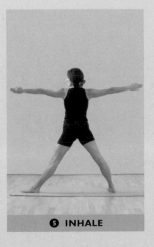

❸ INHALE
❹ EXHALE

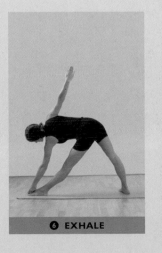

❺ INHALE

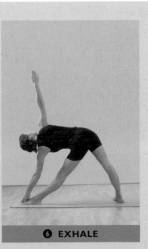

❻ EXHALE

❻ EXHALE

PARIVRTTA TRIKONASANA
REVOLVING TRIANGLE

BENEFITS: This is the first twist. All twists relieve backache, headache, and stiff necks and shoulders. They improve spinal flexibility and open the hips. They also stimulate the digestion by massaging the internal organs.

CONTRAINDICATIONS: NO TWISTING IS PERMITTED DURING PREGNANCY OR AFTER ABDOMINAL SURGERY. SEEK MEDICAL ADVICE IF YOU ARE SUFFERING FROM A HERNIA.

❶ INHALE: Come up from Utthita Trikonasana. Return your feet to parallel position then turn your right foot out 90 degrees as before, this time turning your left foot in 45 degrees. Your heels are still lined up. Turn to bring your face, shoulders, and hips in the direction of your right toes, arms extended.

TIP: It is important to be aware of the position of your rear toes. They should never face away from your front foot as this will put strain on your knee.

❷ EXHALE: Fold at a 90-degree angle over your right leg. Keeping your lower back extended and parallel to the floor, twist through your upper torso to bring your left hand flat on the floor outside your right foot.

TIP: If you cannot bring your hand to the floor outside your foot, try resting your fingertips on the floor to the inside of your foot as a transitional move. If you are very stiff you may wish to place one hand on your front hip and work on keeping your hips squared while you come to a 90-degree angle over your front leg. ONLY begin to twist once the forward bend is complete.

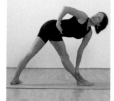

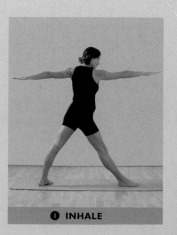

❶ INHALE

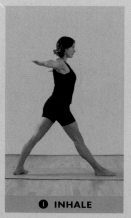

❶ INHALE

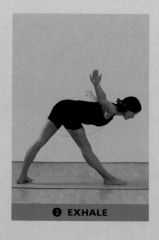

❷ EXHALE

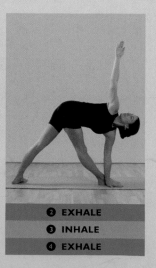

❷ EXHALE
❸ INHALE
❹ EXHALE

❸ INHALE: Bring your right arm vertically in line with your left. Look up at your right thumb.

❹ EXHALE: Hold for 5 breaths.

❺ INHALE: Come up. Keep your arms extended. Switch the position of your feet so that you are facing the opposite direction.

❻ EXHALE: Repeat the posture on the left side.

❼ INHALE: Come up with arms extended and bring your feet back to parallel position.

❽ EXHALE: Jump back to face the front of the mat, bringing your feet together in Neutral Pose.

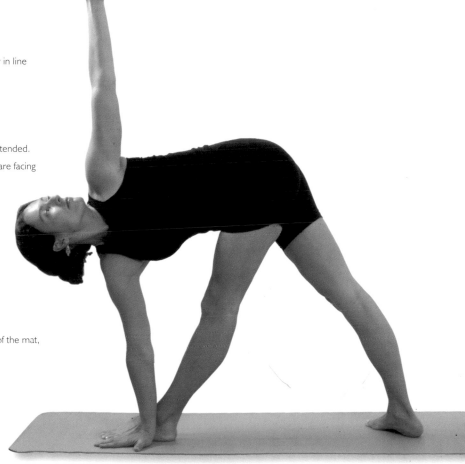

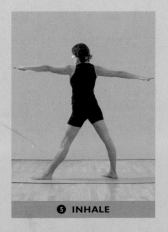
❺ INHALE

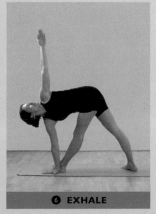
❻ EXHALE

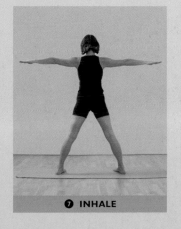
❼ INHALE

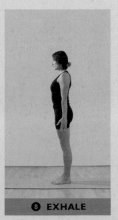
❽ EXHALE

UTTHITA PARSVAKONASANA
LATERAL EXTENSION

BENEFITS: This intense hip and groin opener develops strength in the legs and flexibility in the upper back and shoulders.

❶ INHALE: From Neutral Pose, jump to the right, arms extended to the sides, and feet apart, landing with them parallel under your wrists. Turn your right foot out 90 degrees, keeping your heels lined up.

❷ EXHALE: Bend your right knee to bring it in line with your ankle. Reach beyond your knee with your right arm and place your right hand on the floor outside your right foot.

MODIFICATION
Pregnant women may prefer to rest the elbow on the bent leg rather than bringing the hand to the floor.

❸ INHALE: Reach up vertically with your left arm, opening your chest and bringing your arms and shoulders vertically in line.

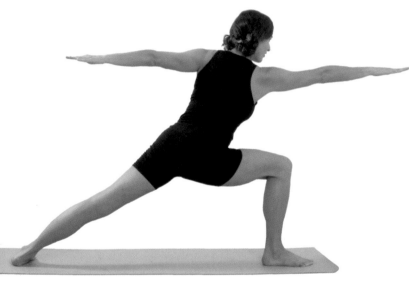

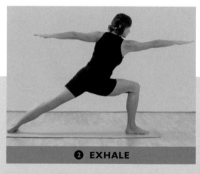

❷ EXHALE

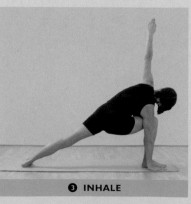

❸ INHALE

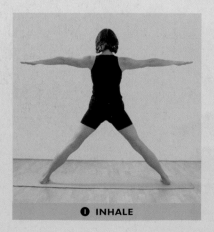

❶ INHALE

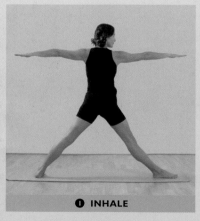

❶ INHALE

TIP: Keep working on bringing your extended arm to vertical before attempting to bring it to 45 degrees. This is a side stretch, so leaning forward or arching your back must be avoided. Good use of bandha and correct placement of your feet will keep your body correctly aligned in all standing postures.

❺ INHALE: Come up, keeping your arms extended. Switch the position of your feet so that you are facing the opposite direction.

❻ EXHALE: Repeat the posture on the left side.

❹ EXHALE: Turn your palm and extend your arm 45 degrees over your head. Look up into your palm. **Hold for 5 breaths.**

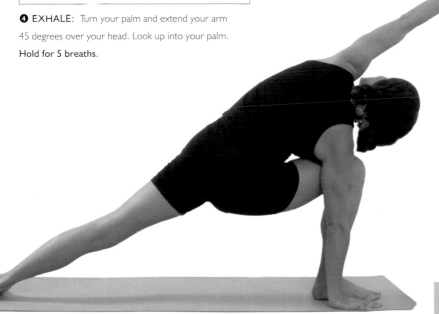

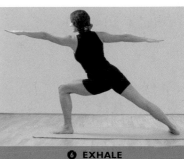

❻ EXHALE

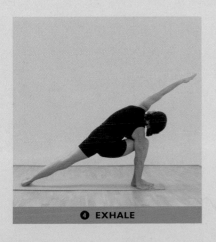

❹ EXHALE

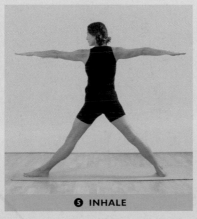

❺ INHALE

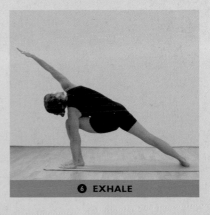

❻ EXHALE

PARIVRTTA PARSVAKONASANA
REVOLVING LATERAL EXTENSION

BENEFITS: This posture builds on the work of the previous postures and encourages the lungs and ribs to expand.

> **CONTRAINDICATIONS**: NO TWISTING IS PERMITTED DURING PREGNANCY OR AFTER ABDOMINAL SURGERY. SEEK MEDICAL ADVICE IF YOU ARE SUFFERING FROM A HERNIA.

❶ INHALE: Come up from Utthita Parsvakonasana. Return your feet to parallel position, then turn your right foot out 90 degrees as before, this time turning your left foot in 45 degrees. Your heels are still lined up. Turn to bring your face, shoulders, and hips in the direction of your right toes.

❷ EXHALE: Bend your right knee and twist to wedge your left arm behind your right leg, bringing your hand to the floor outside your right foot.

❸ INHALE: Reach up vertically with your right arm, opening your chest and shoulders.

❹ EXHALE: Turn your palm to face the floor as you extend your arm over your head. Look into your right palm. **Hold for 5 breaths.**

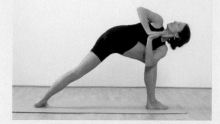

MODIFICATION
Beginners may want to bring the hands together in prayer position in front of the sternum instead of extending the arms.

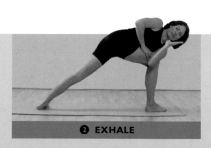

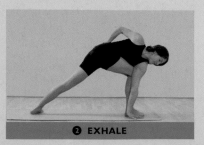

❶ INHALE

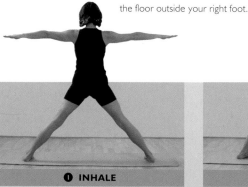

❶ INHALE

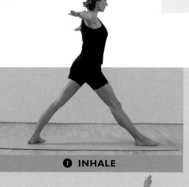

❷ EXHALE

❷ EXHALE

❸ INHALE

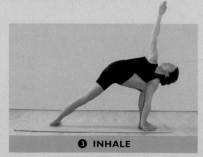

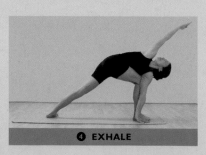

❹ EXHALE

TIP: It can be helpful to work into this posture while kneeling on your back knee but, if you do so, lift your knee and bring your back foot into the correct position before reaching up with your top arm. Work on the posture by squaring your hips, pushing down on the outside edge of your back foot to lift the arch, and bending deeper into your front knee.

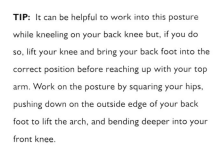

❺ INHALE: Come up, keeping your arms extended. Switch the position of your feet so that you are facing the opposite direction.

❻ EXHALE: Repeat the posture on the left side.

❼ INHALE: Come up with your arms extended to the sides, bringing your feet into parallel position.

❽ EXHALE: Jump back to face the front of the mat, bringing your feet together in Neutral Pose.

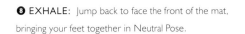

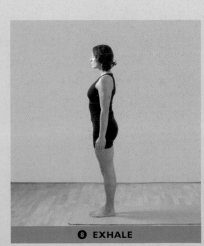

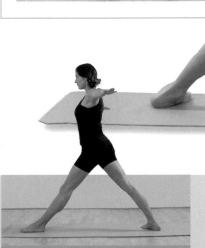

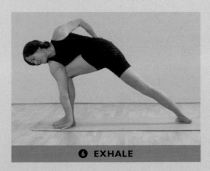

❺ INHALE

❻ EXHALE

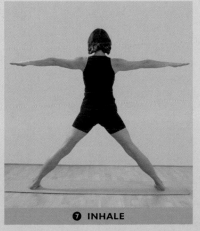

❼ INHALE

❽ EXHALE

PRASARITA PADOTTANASANA A, B, C, AND D
WIDE-LEGGED FORWARD BEND

BENEFITS: This sequence continues to work on the flexibility of the back of the body and shoulders, and encourages bandha practice.

> **CONTRAINDICATIONS:** KEEP HANDS ON THE GROUND WHEN PREGNANT.

❶ INHALE: From Neutral Pose, jump to the right, with your arms extended to the sides and your feet apart, landing with them parallel under your palms. As you land, bring your hands to your waist and draw your shoulders and elbows back to open your chest.

❷ EXHALE: Fold forward, bringing your hands to the floor shoulder distance apart between your feet. Arms are parallel.

❸ INHALE: Look up.

❹ EXHALE: Fold forward to bring your head to the floor between your hands. Look at your nose. **Hold for 5 breaths.**

❺ INHALE: Look up.

❻ EXHALE: Bring your hands to your waist.

❼ INHALE: Come all the way up.

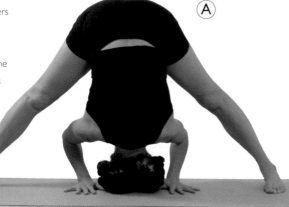

Ⓐ

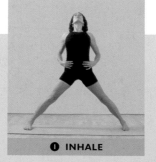

❶ INHALE

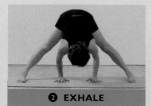

❷ EXHALE

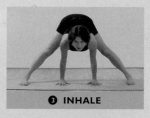

❸ INHALE

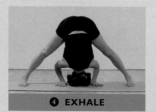

❹ EXHALE

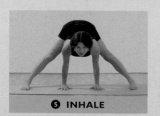

❺ INHALE

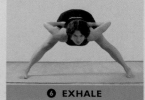

❻ EXHALE

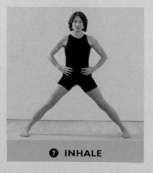

❼ INHALE

❽ EXHALE: Rest your hands on your thighs.

❾ INHALE: Arms out to the sides.

❿ EXHALE: Hands to waist.

⓫ INHALE: Open your chest and shoulders.

⓬ EXHALE: Fold forward, keeping your hands on your waist and bringing your head to the floor between your feet. Look at your nose. **Hold for 5 breaths.**

> ### MODIFICATION
> When pregnant you may want to walk your hands down a wall or bend your knees to support your hands and work on extending your spine.

⓭ INHALE: Come all the way up, keeping your hands on your waist.

⓮ EXHALE: Rest your hands on your thighs.

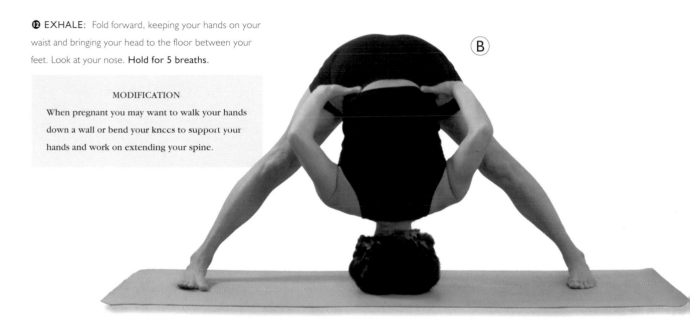

B

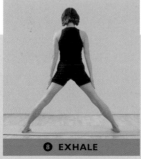

❽ EXHALE

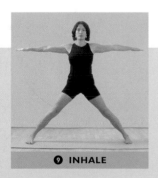

❾ INHALE

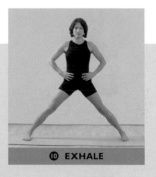

❿ EXHALE

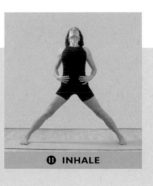

⓫ INHALE

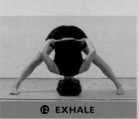

⓬ EXHALE

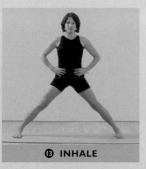

⓭ INHALE

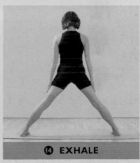

⓮ EXHALE

⓯ INHALE: Bring your arms out to the sides.

⓰ EXHALE: Lace your fingers together behind your back. If possible turn your palms to face out.

⓱ INHALE: Straighten your arms and open your shoulders and chest.

⓲ EXHALE: Come forward to bring your head to the floor between your feet and your hands to the floor over the top of your head. Look at your nose. **Hold for 5 breaths.**

⓳ INHALE: Come all the way up, keeping your hands behind your back.

⓴ EXHALE: Rest your hands on your waist.

㉑ INHALE: Open your chest.

C

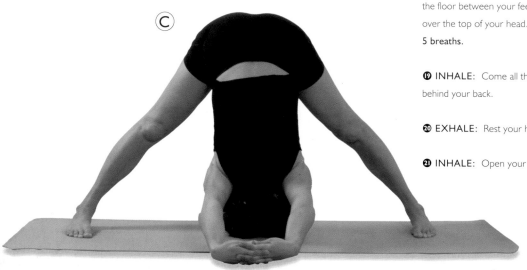

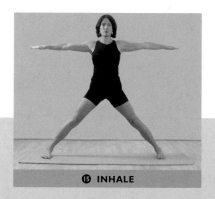

⓯ INHALE

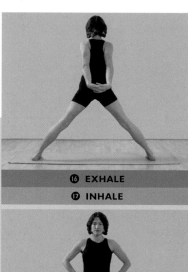

⓰ EXHALE
⓱ INHALE

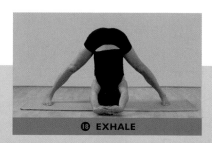

⓲ EXHALE

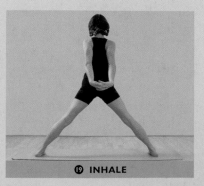

⓳ INHALE

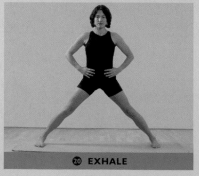

⓴ EXHALE

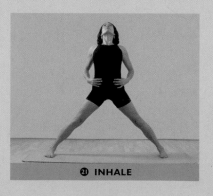

㉑ INHALE

22 EXHALE: Fold forward and grab your big toes

23 INHALE: Look up.

24 EXHALE: Bring your head to the floor. Look at your nose. **Hold for 5 breaths.**

25 INHALE: Look up, keeping the toe grip.

26 EXHALE: Hands to waist.

27 INHALE: Come all the way up, keeping your hands on your waist.

28 EXHALE: Jump back to Neutral Pose, landing with your feet together facing the front of the mat, arms by your sides.

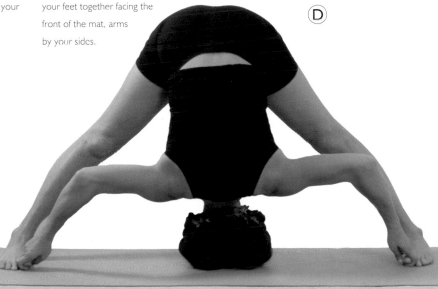

(D)

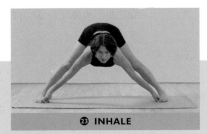

22 EXHALE

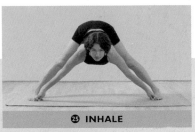

23 INHALE

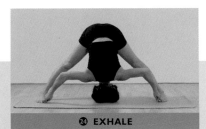

24 EXHALE

25 INHALE

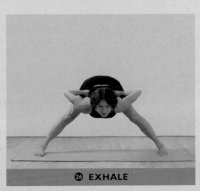

26 EXHALE

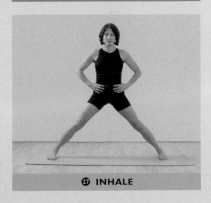

27 INHALE

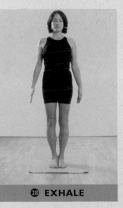

28 EXHALE

PARSVOTTANASANA
LATERAL FORWARD BEND

BENEFITS: This forward bend opens the shoulders, straightens the spine, and stretches the pectoral area to improve circulation and tone the muscles supporting the breasts.

❶ INHALE: From Neutral Pose, jump to the right, arms extended and feet apart. Land with your feet parallel under your elbows. Turn your right foot out 90 degrees, then turn your left foot in 45 degrees. Heels are lined up. Turn to face in the direction of your right toes, arms extended, shoulders in line, hips in line.

❷ EXHALE: Bring your arms behind your back and place your hands in prayer position with your fingers pointing up your spine, palms together.

MODIFICATION

If it is impossible even to begin bringing your hands into prayer position, try holding your elbows behind your back as a transitional modification. Keep working your shoulders back to open your chest.

❸ INHALE: Open your chest and shoulders and press your palms together.

❹ EXHALE: Fold forward over your right leg. Look at your right foot. **Hold for 5 breaths.**

❺ INHALE: Come up, keeping your arms together behind your back.

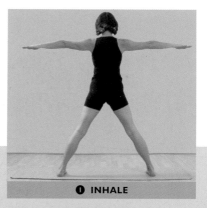
❶ INHALE

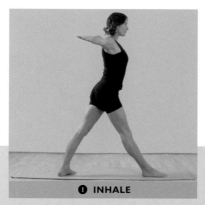
❶ INHALE

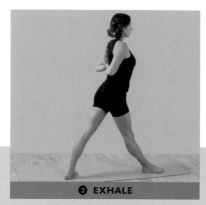
❷ EXHALE

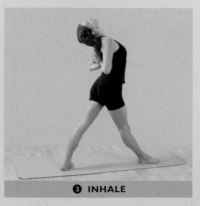
❸ INHALE

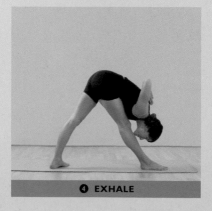
❹ EXHALE

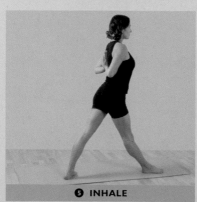
❺ INHALE

❻ EXHALE: Switch the position of your feet and repeat on the left.

❼ INHALE: Come up, bringing your feet back to parallel position.

❽ EXHALE: Jump back to Neutral Pose, facing the front of the mat, with your feet together.

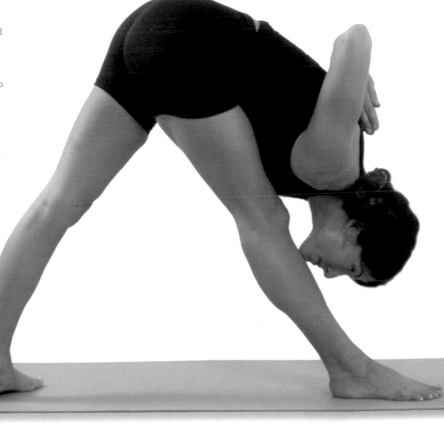

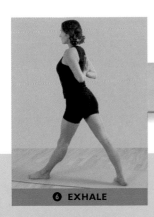

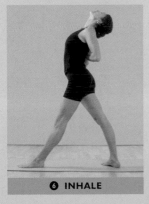

❻ EXHALE

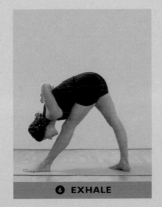

❻ INHALE

❻ EXHALE

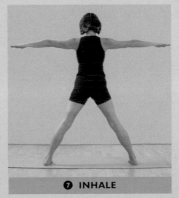

❼ INHALE

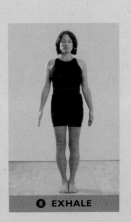

❽ EXHALE

UTTHITA HASTA PADANGUSTHASANA
EXTENDED LEG BALANCES

BENEFITS: Leg Balances improve strength, flexibility, balance, and bandha control.

> **CONTRAINDICATIONS**: WHEN PREGNANT, HOLD YOUR KNEE RATHER THAN YOUR TOE (SEE TIP), AS EXTENDING YOUR LEG MAY CAUSE STRAIN IN YOUR LOWER BACK.

❶ INHALE: Balance on your left foot with your left hand on your waist. Hold your right big toe with the first two fingers and thumb of your right hand and extend your leg as high as possible.

❷ EXHALE: Draw your chin to your shin. Look at your foot. **Hold for 5 breaths.**

❸ INHALE: Stand up straight.

❹ EXHALE: Bring your right leg out to the right, turning your gaze and your head to the left. **Hold for 5 breaths.**

MODIFICATION

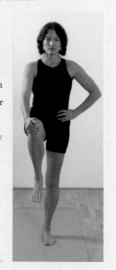

If you have very tight hips and hamstrings, you may need to hold your knee rather than your toe in this position and when bringing your leg out to the side. If this is the case, you may also find it helpful to repeat the standing postures rather than moving foward in the Primary Series. This modificiation can also be used when pregnant.

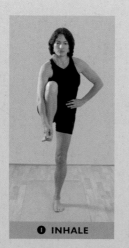
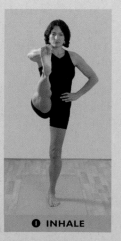
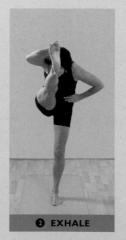
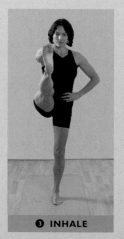
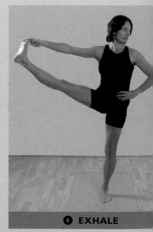

❶ INHALE   ❶ INHALE   ❷ EXHALE   ❸ INHALE   ❹ EXHALE

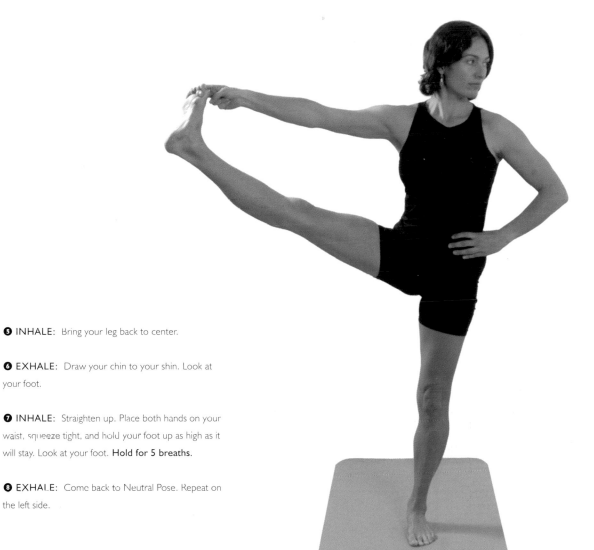

❺ INHALE: Bring your leg back to center.

❻ EXHALE: Draw your chin to your shin. Look at your foot.

❼ INHALE: Straighten up. Place both hands on your waist, squeeze tight, and hold your foot up as high as it will stay. Look at your foot. **Hold for 5 breaths.**

❽ EXHALE: Come back to Neutral Pose. Repeat on the left side.

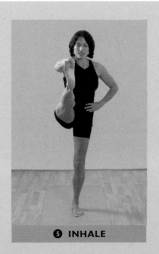

❺ INHALE

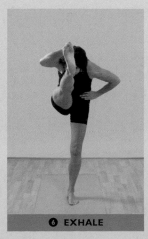

❻ EXHALE

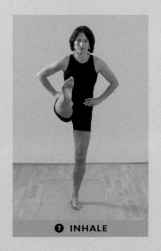

❼ INHALE

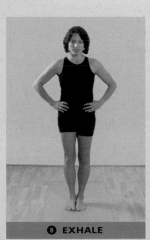

❽ EXHALE

ARDHA BADDHA PADMOTTANASANA
STANDING HALF-BOUND LOTUS FORWARD BEND

BENEFITS: This sequence can ease PMS and sciatica,* and improves circulation to the spleen and liver.

CONTRAINDICATIONS: WHEN PREGNANT DO NOT FOLD FORWARD. PERFORM WITH CARE IF SUFFERING FROM KNEE PROBLEMS.

❶ INHALE: Balance on your left foot and bring your right leg into Half Lotus.

❷ (EXHALE:) Reach behind your back and clasp your foot with your right hand.

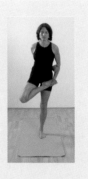

MODIFICATION
If you are stiff in the hips or have pain in your knees, start by bringing your knee into your chest and balancing there before or instead of working into Lotus position. If you cannot clasp your foot hold your forearm instead.

❸ (INHALE:) Stand up straight, aligning your shoulders and hips.

❹ EXHALE: Fold forward, bringing your left hand to the floor outside your left foot.

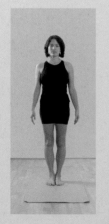

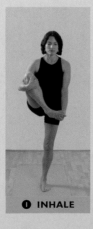
❶ INHALE

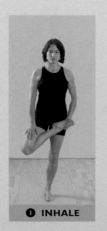
❶ INHALE

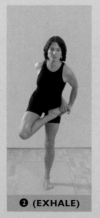
❷ (EXHALE)

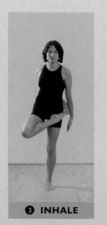
❸ INHALE

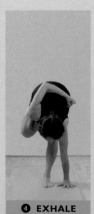
❹ EXHALE

❺ INHALE: Extend your spine. Look up.

❻ EXHALE: Bring your chin to your shin. Look at your foot. **Hold for 5 breaths.**

❼ INHALE: Look up.

❽ EXHALE: Hold the position and bend your standing leg slightly.

❾ INHALE: Come up.

❿ EXHALE: Release to Neutral Pose. Repeat on the left side then come back to Neutral Pose at the front of the mat.

> *** NOTE ABOUT SCIATICA:** INCORRECT FORWARD BENDING CAN AGGRAVATE THIS CONDITION. PROCEED WITH CARE. ALWAYS SEE A MEDICAL PROFESSIONAL IF YOU SUSPECT YOU SUFFER FROM SCIATICA.

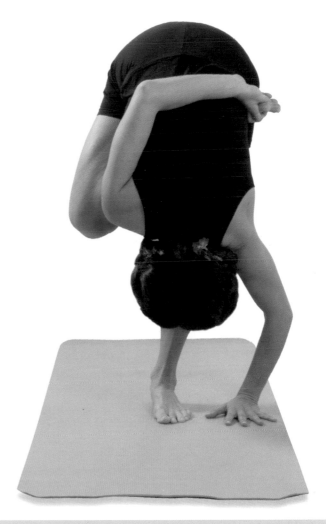

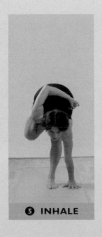
❺ INHALE

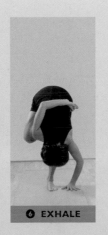
❻ EXHALE

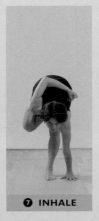
❼ INHALE

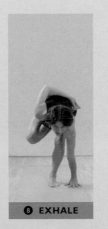
❽ EXHALE

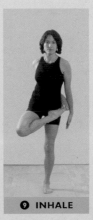
❾ INHALE

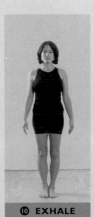
❿ EXHALE

THE WARRIOR SEQUENCE

BENEFITS: The Warrior Sequence combines the asanas of the two Sun Salutations. Holding Utkatasana and the Warrior Postures rather than flowing through them increases the strength of the spine, arms, and legs.

UTKATASANA
SEAT OF POWER

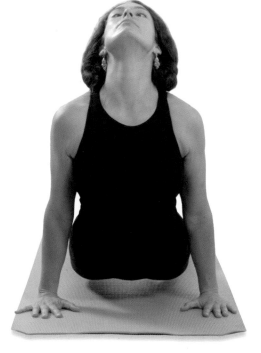

❶ INHALE: Reach up with straight arms, bringing your palms together. Look up at your thumbs.

❷ EXHALE: Fold forward from your hips, bring your hands to the floor shoulder distance apart, and tuck in your head. Look at your nose.

❸ INHALE: Lift your head to open your chest and extend the spine. Look up.

❹ EXHALE: Jump back, feet hip distance apart, to a push-up position. Bend your elbows and bring your chin two inches from the floor, keeping your chest, pelvis, and knees off the floor. Look at your nose.

❺ INHALE: Push your chest forward, straighten your arms, and roll over your toes to Upward Dog. Look at your nose.

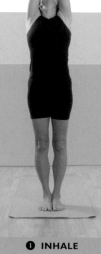
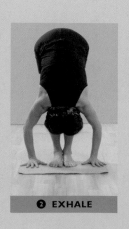
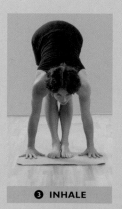
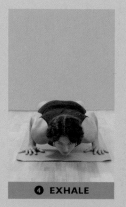
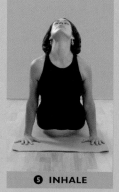

❶ INHALE   ❷ EXHALE   ❸ INHALE   ❹ EXHALE   ❺ INHALE

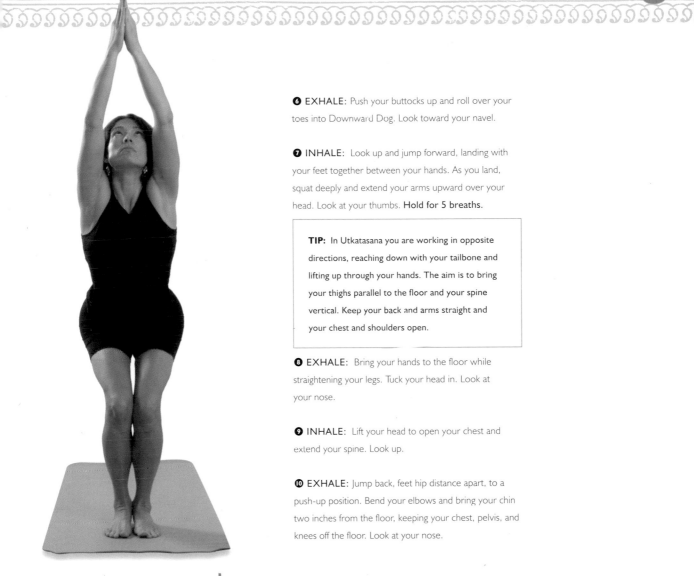

❻ EXHALE: Push your buttocks up and roll over your toes into Downward Dog. Look toward your navel.

❼ INHALE: Look up and jump forward, landing with your feet together between your hands. As you land, squat deeply and extend your arms upward over your head. Look at your thumbs. **Hold for 5 breaths.**

> **TIP:** In Utkatasana you are working in opposite directions, reaching down with your tailbone and lifting up through your hands. The aim is to bring your thighs parallel to the floor and your spine vertical. Keep your back and arms straight and your chest and shoulders open.

❽ EXHALE: Bring your hands to the floor while straightening your legs. Tuck your head in. Look at your nose.

❾ INHALE: Lift your head to open your chest and extend your spine. Look up.

❿ EXHALE: Jump back, feet hip distance apart, to a push-up position. Bend your elbows and bring your chin two inches from the floor, keeping your chest, pelvis, and knees off the floor. Look at your nose.

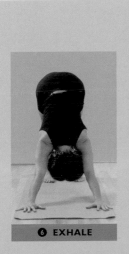

❻ EXHALE

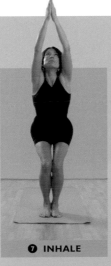

❼ INHALE

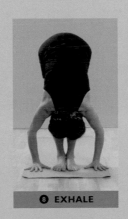

❽ EXHALE

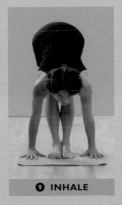

❾ INHALE

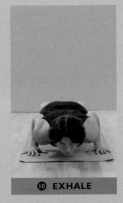

❿ EXHALE

THE PRIMARY SERIES

VIRABHADRASANA A AND B
WARRIOR POSTURES

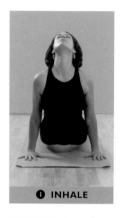

❶ INHALE

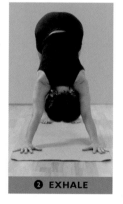

❷ EXHALE

❶ INHALE: Push your chest forward, straighten your arms, and roll over your toes into Upward Dog. Look at your nose.

❷ EXHALE: Push your buttocks up and roll over your toes into Downward Dog. Before the end of the exhalation, turn the heel of your left foot toward the ball of your right foot and step your right foot between your hands. Keep your heels on the floor and in line. Your front leg is bent 90 degrees so your knee is directly above your ankle. Your back leg is straight.

❸ INHALE: Reach up, bringing your palms together. Your arms and spine are vertical, your hips and shoulders face evenly forward. Look up at your thumbs.

> **MODIFICATION**
> If pregnant keep your hands on your hips
> to avoid straining your sacroiliac joint.

❹ EXHALE: Hold for 5 breaths.

❺ INHALE: Straighten your right leg. Come up, keeping your arms up. Turn your right toes in and your left toes out.

❻ EXHALE: Bend your left leg, move into the posture as on the right. Look at your thumbs. **Hold for 5 breaths.**

❼ INHALE: Prepare to change position.

❽ EXHALE: Extend your arms in line with your body and take your rear toes to 90 degrees, allowing your right hip and shoulder to open out 90 degrees to the side. Your left leg remains bent with your knee directly over your ankle. Keep your spine vertical. Look at your left hand. **Hold for 5 breaths.**

❾ INHALE: Come up and change sides.

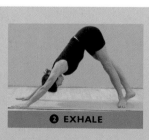

❷ EXHALE

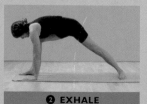

❷ EXHALE

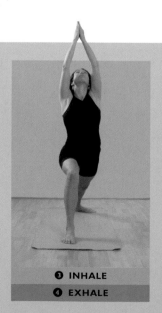

❸ INHALE
❹ EXHALE

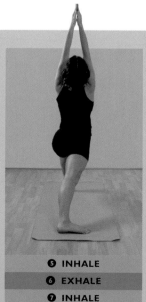

❺ INHALE
❻ EXHALE
❼ INHALE

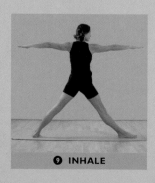

❽ EXHALE

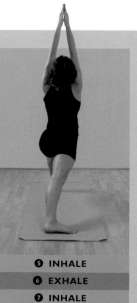

❾ INHALE

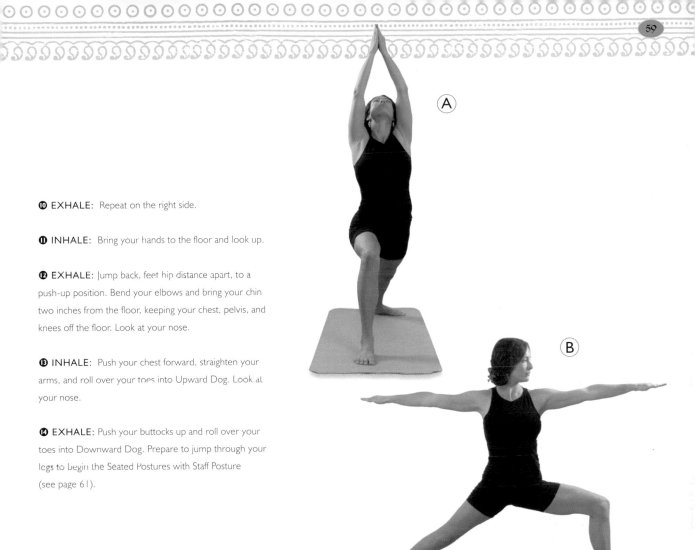

A

B

❿ EXHALE: Repeat on the right side.

⓫ INHALE: Bring your hands to the floor and look up.

⓬ EXHALE: Jump back, feet hip distance apart, to a push-up position. Bend your elbows and bring your chin two inches from the floor, keeping your chest, pelvis, and knees off the floor. Look at your nose.

⓭ INHALE: Push your chest forward, straighten your arms, and roll over your toes into Upward Dog. Look at your nose.

⓮ EXHALE: Push your buttocks up and roll over your toes into Downward Dog. Prepare to jump through your legs to begin the Seated Postures with Staff Posture (see page 61).

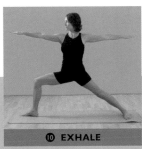

❿ EXHALE

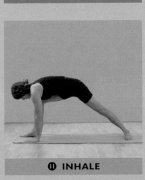

⓫ INHALE

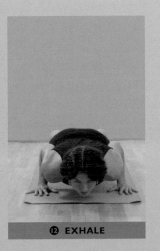

⓬ EXHALE

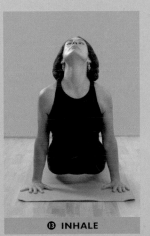

⓭ INHALE

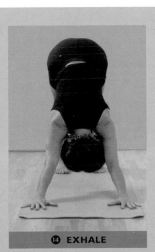

⓮ EXHALE

THE SITTING POSTURES
(THE PRIMARY SERIES)
YOGA CHIKITSA – YOGA THERAPY

Having warmed the muscles and stilled the mind with
the Sun Salutations and Standing Postures, the body
should now be ready for the Primary Series. Again,
these postures are practiced in a specific order and can
be very challenging.

   The keys to mastering the Sitting Postures are
dedication and patience. The Primary Series is powerful
yoga therapy. Work safely with the breath and
awareness, and do not attempt to take the postures
out of sequence.

   The following section describes the Primary Series
as it is most usually taught in groups by Guruji, and
as such may differ slightly in minor details from
information found in other books, classes, or individual
instruction by Guruji. This is not a "full Vinyasa
practice," but is the most common form. In particular,
the correct breath sequence has been observed, with
optional extra breaths and movements suggested
in parenthesis. The Primary Series postures should be
mastered before attempting those of the Intermediate
or Advanced series.

DANDASANA
STAFF POSTURE

BENEFITS: Staff Posture prepares the body for correct forward bending by lengthening the spine and the back of the legs.

❶ INHALE: From Downward Dog, jump your feet through your hands and sit down with your legs straight in front of you and your feet together.

❷ EXHALE: Keeping your hands on the floor on either side of your hips, with your back vertical, pull back your toes, and pull up on your kneecaps and thighs to strengthen your knees. Look at your toes. **Hold for 5 breaths.**

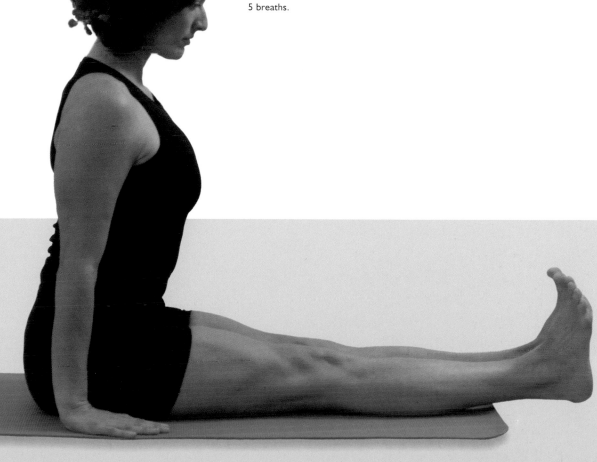

PASCHIMOTTANASANA
SEATED FORWARD BEND

BENEFITS: Seated Forward Bend helps relieve sciatica, shin splints, prolapsed uterus, and menopausal symptoms. It stills the mind, and is also good during menstruation.

❶ INHALE: Open your shoulders and chest.

❷ EXHALE: Lean forward and grasp your big toes with the first two fingers and thumbs of each hand.

❸ INHALE: Lengthen your torso.

❹ EXHALE: Fold forward, keeping the front and back of your body long. Look toward your feet.
Hold for 5 breaths.

TIP: In this and all subsequent forward bends, work your belly to your thighs, chest to your knees, and chin between your shins. Do not drop your head prematurely. Uddiyana Bandha will support and lengthen your spine.

MODIFICATION
If you cannot reach your big toes, it may be beneficial to go back to the beginning of the Standing Postures and work on them rather than going forward into the Primary Series. Pregnant women may need to open their legs in forward bends to allow space for the baby.

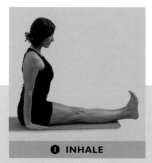
❶ INHALE

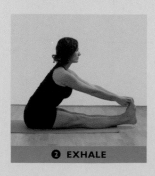
❷ EXHALE

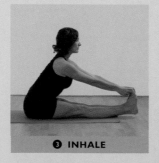
❸ INHALE

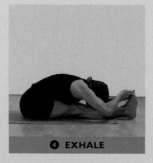
❹ EXHALE

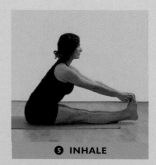
❺ INHALE

❺ INHALE: Look up, keeping your grip on your toes.

❻ EXHALE: Lock your hands around your feet, holding your wrist if possible.

❼ INHALE: Look up and lift your chest.

❽ EXHALE: Fold down again. Look at your feet.
Hold for 5 breaths.

❾ INHALE: Look up.

❿ EXHALE: Release your hands to the floor forward of your hips.

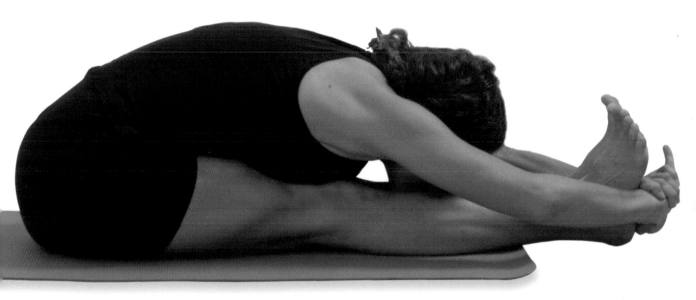

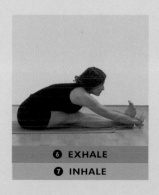

❻ EXHALE
❼ INHALE

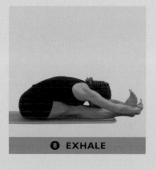

❽ EXHALE

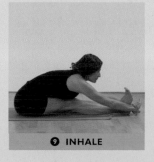

❾ INHALE

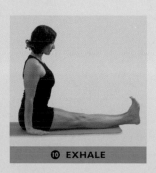

❿ EXHALE

VINYASA
LINKING MOVEMENTS

The Seated Postures are linked by a sequence of moves known as a Vinyasa that neutralizes the body between postures and keeps it warm. In this chapter we describe the most commonly used "Half Vinyasa" that should be used after releasing each posture.

> **TIP:** Lifting is difficult for women because of their low center of gravity but with persistence it is possible to develop the strength to lift your back and jump through in the Vinyasas. It is best to attempt to lift in every Vinyasa but at first your feet may have to be dragged through your hands or it may be necessary to roll forward on to your hands and knees before jumping back.

❶ INHALE: Cross your legs and lift your buttocks and feet off the ground.

❷ EXHALE: Jump back, feet hip distance apart, to a push-up position. Bend your elbows and bring your chin one inch from the floor, keeping your chest, pelvis, and knees off the floor. Look at your nose.

❸ INHALE: Push your chest forward, straighten your arms, and roll over your toes into Upward Dog. Look at your nose.

❹ EXHALE: Push your buttocks up and roll over your toes into Downward Dog.

❺ INHALE: Jump your feet through your hands and sit down.

> **TIP:** There are two ways of jumping through. If you jump through with legs crossed, remember to look up to get lift and use bandha control. To jump through with straight legs, imagine that you are jumping to standing, just don't stop. If you cannot jump through, jump your feet to your hands and sit down from there.

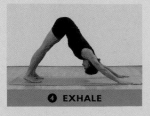
❶ INHALE

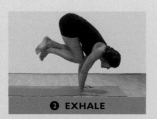
❷ EXHALE

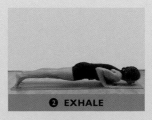
❷ EXHALE

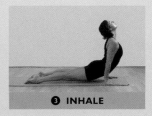
❸ INHALE

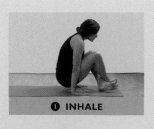
❹ EXHALE

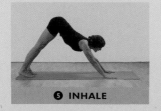
❺ INHALE

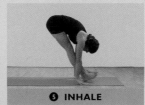
❺ INHALE

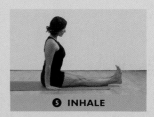
❺ INHALE

PURVOTTANASANA
SEATED BACK BEND

BENEFITS: This counterpose to the Forward Bend tones the reproductive organs.

> ### MODIFICATION
> If pregnant, perform with bent knees to avoid straining your back.

❶ INHALE: Jump your feet through your hands and sit down with your legs straight and feet together.

❷ EXHALE: Bring your hands to the floor one foot away from your buttocks, fingers pointing forward. Point your toes.

❸ INHALE: Lift your pelvis, abdomen, and chest, keeping your legs straight. Drop your head back and look at your nose. **Hold for 5 breaths.**

❹ EXHALE: Release. Bring your hands to the floor in front of your hips.

❺ INHALE: Do your Vinyasa.

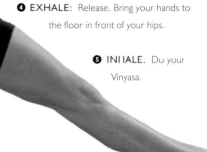

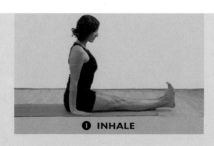

❶ INHALE

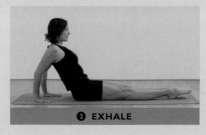

❷ EXHALE

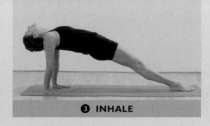

❸ INHALE

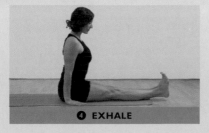

❹ EXHALE

ARDHA BADDHA PADMA PASCHIMOTTANASANA
SEATED HALF-BOUND LOTUS FORWARD BEND

BENEFITS: This eases sciatica, and massages the liver and spleen.

> **CONTRAINDICATIONS:** IF PREGNANT, DO NOT FOLD FORWARD.

❶ **INHALE:** Jump your feet through your hands and sit down with your legs straight. (EXHALE:) Bring your right foot into Half Lotus, and clasp your foot with your right hand. (INHALE:) Reach for your left foot with your left hand. Look up.

❷ **EXHALE:** Fold forward, bringing your chin to your left shin, and look at your left toes. **Hold for 5 breaths.**

❸ **INHALE:** Look up.

❹ **EXHALE:** Release. Bring your hands to the floor in front of your hips.

❺ **INHALE:** Do your Vinyasa. Repeat on the left side.

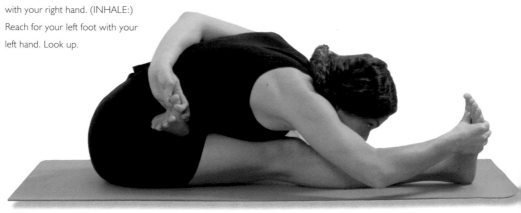

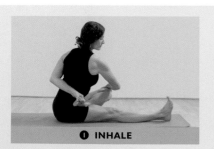

❶ INHALE

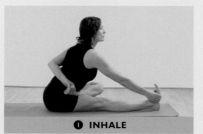

❶ INHALE

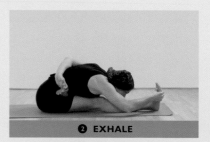

❷ EXHALE

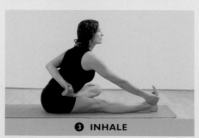

❸ INHALE

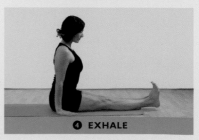

❹ EXHALE

TIRIANGMUKHAIKAPADA PASCHIMOTTANASANA
TRANSVERSE BENT KNEE FORWARD BEND

BENEFITS: The intense stretch in the buttocks and lower back can be helpful with sciatica. This Forward Bend also opens the hips.

❶ INHALE: As you jump through from your Vinyasa, bend your right shin under and land with your left leg extended, knees together, and your right foot pointing backward outside your right hip. The sole of your right foot faces up to prevent knee strain. Hold your left wrist with your right hand around your left foot.

> **TIP:** Stiff hips can put pressure on the knees in this posture. Be careful. If necessary do not come forward. Support yourself with your hands on the floor on either side of your hips, and work on the position of your legs.

❷ EXHALE: Fold forward over your left leg, taking your chin to your left shin. Look at your left foot. **Hold for 5 breaths.**

> **MODIFICATION**
> Pregnant women should work on creating space in the torso and may want to use a belt around the extended foot to lift and open into the posture rather than folding forward in this and subsequent postures.

❸ INHALE: Look up.

❹ EXHALE: Release. Bring your hands to the floor in front of your hips.

❺ INHALE: Do your Vinyasa. Repeat on the left side.

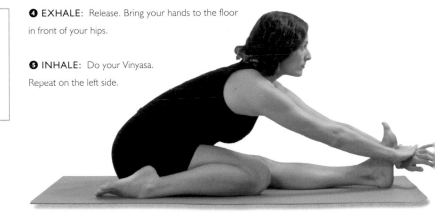

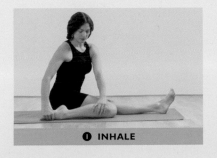

❶ INHALE

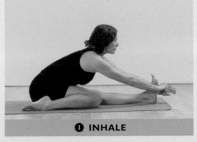

❶ INHALE

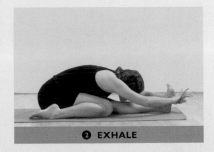

❷ EXHALE

JANU SIRSASANA A
BENT KNEE FORWARD BEND A

BENEFITS: This posture is beneficial during menstruation. It helps a prolapsed uterus, relieves symptoms of cystitis, and opens the hips.

❶ INHALE: Jump through from your Vinyasa, (EXHALE:) bend your right leg, bringing your right heel to your groin and your knee 90 degrees out to the side. (INHALE:) Lock your hands around your left foot and extend your spine, aligning your shoulders and hips.

❷ EXHALE: Fold forward from your hips, look at your left foot. **Hold for 5 breaths.**

❸ INHALE: Look up.

❹ EXHALE: Release. Bring your hands to the floor in front of your hips.

❺ INHALE: Do your Vinyasa. Repeat on the left side.

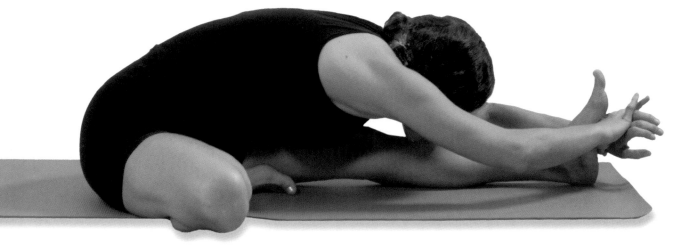

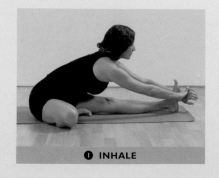
❶ INHALE

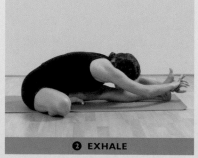
❷ EXHALE

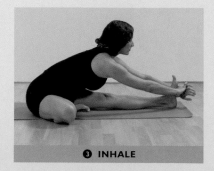
❸ INHALE

JANU SIRSASANA B
BENT KNEE FORWARD BEND B

BENEFITS: This is good for stretching and strengthening the ankles. It encourages the practice of Mula Bandha. It is also helpful for toning the pelvic floor and prolapsed uterus.

❶ INHALE: Jump through from your Vinyasa. (EXHALE:) Bend your right leg, bringing your right heel under your groin and your knee 85 degrees out to the side. (INHALE:) Lift your buttocks off the ground. (EXHALE:) Sit your anus on your heel. (INHALE:) Lock your hands around your left foot and extend your spine, aligning your shoulders and hips.

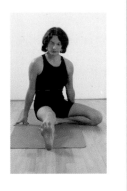

> TIP: Beginners work into Janu Sirsasana A first, then lift the buttocks to sit the anus on the heel. At first the toes of the bent leg may need to point out to the side rather than forward.

❷ EXHALE: Fold forward from your hips. Look at your left foot. Hold for 5 breaths.

> TIP: This posture may cause discomfort in the ankle you are sitting on. Use a towel for padding until you toughen up. In some cases this posture can cause pressure in the knees. Work gently if this is the case.

❸ INHALE: Look up.

❹ EXHALE: Release. Bring your hands to the floor in front of your hips.

❺ INHALE: Do your Vinyasa. Repeat on the left side.

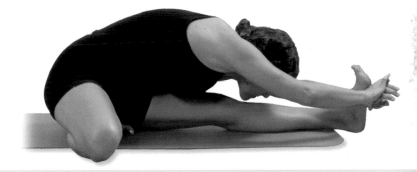

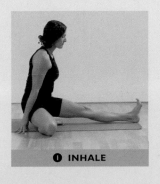

❶ INHALE

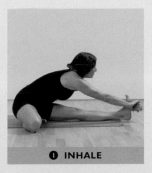

❶ INHALE

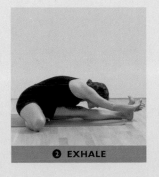

❷ EXHALE

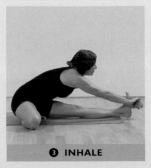

❸ INHALE

JANU SIRSASANA C
BENT KNEE FORWARD BEND C

BENEFITS: This is useful for massaging and toning the uterus. It may encourage the breakdown of fibroids and ease other uterine difficulties, and it stimulates the pancreas.

> **CONTRAINDICATIONS:** DO NOT PRACTICE IF PREGNANT.

❶ INHALE: Jump through from the linking movement. (EXHALE:) Bend your right leg and hold your heel with your left hand. Reach through to grasp the front of your foot with your right hand and keep your heel lifted as you place the ball of your foot on the floor in tiptoe position, pointing away from your left thigh in front of your groin. Lower your right knee to the floor. (INHALE:) Lock your hands around your left foot and extend your spine, aligning your shoulders and hips. Try to bring your right heel into your navel.

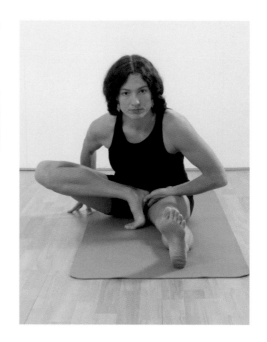

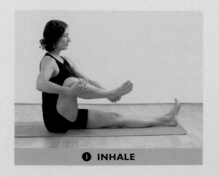

❶ INHALE

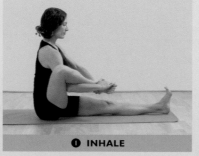

❶ INHALE

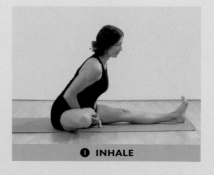

❶ INHALE

TIP: To work deeper into the foot position, you can place your hands on the floor either side of your hips and on an inhalation lift your body to bring your weight forward into your toe.

❷ **EXHALE:** Fold forward from your hips and look at your left foot. **Hold for 5 breaths.**

❸ INHALE: Look up.

❹ **EXHALE:** Release. Bring your hands to the floor in front of your hips.

❺ **INHALE:** Do your Vinyasa. Repeat on the left side.

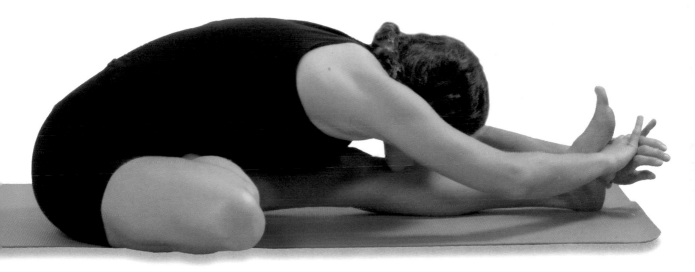

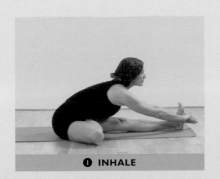

❶ INHALE

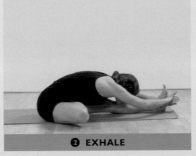

❷ EXHALE

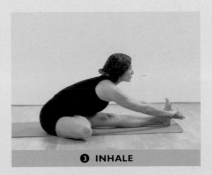

❸ INHALE

MARICHYASANA A
POSTURE OF THE SAGE A

BENEFITS: All the Marichyasana postures are beneficial to the digestive system and the reproductive system. They open the hips and prepare for leg-behind-the-head postures.

❶ INHALE: Jump through with your left leg straight, bend your right leg vertically, and bring your foot flat on the floor so your ankle and the outside of your left hip are lined up. (EXHALE:) Fold forward with your right arm extended and wrap your arm around your right shin, reaching to clasp your left wrist behind your back. (INHALE:) Extend your spine and push back your shoulders.

❷ EXHALE: Fold forward, drawing your chin to your left shin, and look at your left foot. **Hold for 5 breaths.**

❸ INHALE: Look up.

❹ EXHALE: Release. Bring your hands to the floor in front of your hips.

❺ INHALE: Do your Vinyasa. Repeat on the left side. Keeping your knee bent to lift is an advanced option.

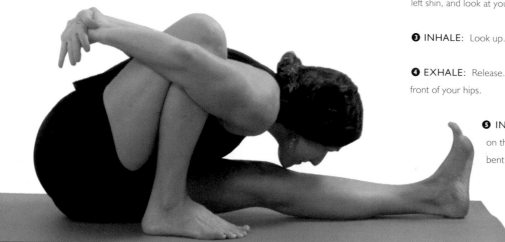

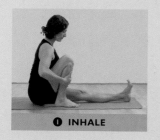

❶ INHALE

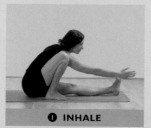

❶ INHALE

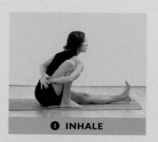

❶ INHALE

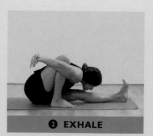

❷ EXHALE

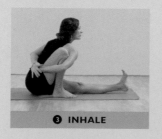

❸ INHALE

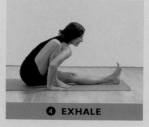

❹ EXHALE

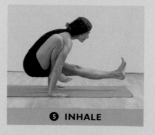

❺ INHALE

MARICHYASANA B
POSTURE OF THE SAGE B

BENEFITS: Regular practice of this posture will strengthen the uterus and may prevent painful menstruation.

CONTRAINDICATIONS: DO NOT PRACTICE THE FULL POSTURE WHEN PREGNANT. IT MAY BE UNSUITABLE DURING MENSTRUATION.

❶ **INHALE:** Jump through with both legs straight. (EXHALE:) Bring your left foot into Lotus. Bend your right leg vertically and bring your foot flat on to the floor so your ankle and the outside of your left hip are lined up. (INHALE:) Lean to the left, lifting your right buttock off the ground and bringing your left knee down, and sit up straight. (EXHALE:) Fold forward with your right arm extended and wrap your arm around your right shin, reaching to clasp your left wrist behind your back. (INHALE:) Extend your spine and push your shoulders back.

MODIFICATION
Pregnant women should avoid pressure in the abdomen, so bring the foot that would normally be in Lotus position to the floor in front of the opposite buttock instead or just repeat the previous posture.

❷ **EXHALE:** Fold forward, drawing your chin to the floor between your foot and knee. Look at your nose. **Hold for 5 breaths.**

❸ **INHALE:** Look up.

❹ **EXHALE:** Release. Bring your hands to the floor in front of your hips.

❺ **INHALE:** Do your Vinyasa. Repeat on the left side.

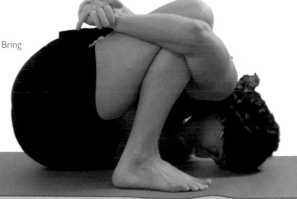

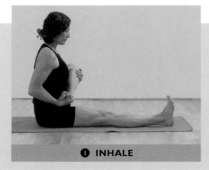
❶ INHALE

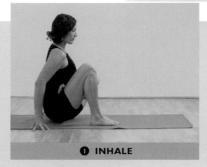
❶ INHALE

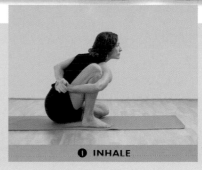
❶ INHALE

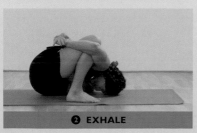
❷ EXHALE

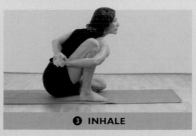
❸ INHALE

MARICHYASANA C
POSTURE OF THE SAGE C

BENEFITS: Twists relieve backache, headache, stiff necks, and tight shoulders. They improve spinal flexibility and open the hips. They stimulate the digestion by massaging the internal organs. Breathing under pressure helps expand the lungs.

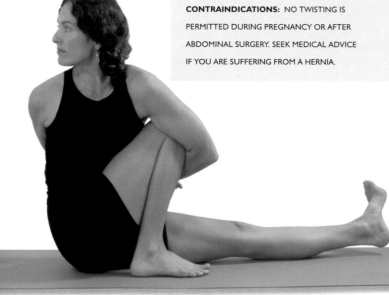

CONTRAINDICATIONS: NO TWISTING IS PERMITTED DURING PREGNANCY OR AFTER ABDOMINAL SURGERY. SEEK MEDICAL ADVICE IF YOU ARE SUFFERING FROM A HERNIA.

❶ INHALE: Jump through with your left leg straight, bend your right leg vertically, and bring your foot flat on the floor so your ankle and the outside of your left hip are lined up. (EXHALE:) Twist to the right, wedge your left upper arm behind your knee and wrap your arm around your right shin, reaching to clasp your right wrist behind your back. (INHALE:) Extend your spine and push back your shoulders.

❷ EXHALE: Twist to the left. Look behind you. **Hold for 5 breaths.**

TIP: Don't lean back when working into the posture—the aim is to straighten your lower back and twist your thoracic spine.

❸ INHALE: Look forward.

❹ EXHALE: Release. Bring your hands to the floor in front of your hips.

❺ INHALE: Do your Vinyasa. Repeat on the left side.

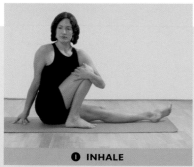
❶ INHALE

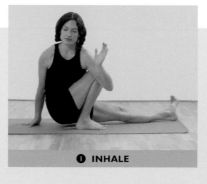
❶ INHALE

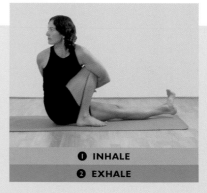
❶ INHALE
❷ EXHALE

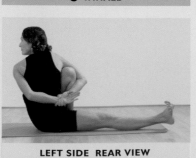
LEFT SIDE REAR VIEW

MARICHYASANA D
POSTURE OF THE SAGE D

BENEFITS: As opposite.

> **CONTRAINDICATIONS:** NO TWISTING IS
> PERMITTED DURING PREGNANCY OR AFTER
> ABDOMINAL SURGERY. SEEK MEDICAL ADVICE
> IF YOU ARE SUFFERING FROM A HERNIA.

> **TIP:** This is a challenging posture, and you may
> need to be adjusted by a teacher to make
> progress. This is also a gateway posture; you
> should be able to get into Marichyasana D before
> attempting to learn the postures after Navasana.

❶ INHALE: Jump through with both legs straight.
(EXHALE:) Bring your left foot into Lotus. Bend your right
leg vertically and place your foot flat on the floor so your
ankle and the outside of your left hip are lined up.
(INHALE:) Lean to the left, lifting your right buttock off
the ground, bringing your left knee down and sit up
straight. (EXHALE:) Twist to the right, wedge your left
upper arm behind your knee, and wrap your arm around
your right shin, reaching to clasp your right wrist behind
your back. (INHALE:) Extend your spine and push your
shoulders back.

❷ EXHALE: Twist to the left. Look behind you.
Hold for 5 breaths.

❸ INHALE: Look forward.

❹ EXHALE: Release. Bring your hands
to the floor in front of your hips.

❺ INHALE: Do your Vinyasa.
Repeat on the left side.

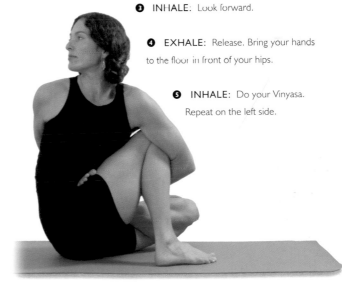

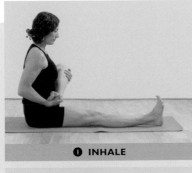

❶ INHALE

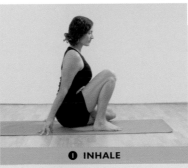

❶ INHALE

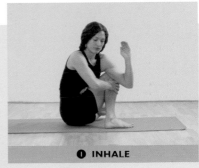

❶ INHALE

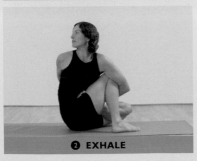

❷ EXHALE

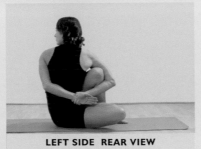

LEFT SIDE REAR VIEW

THE PRIMARY SERIES

NAVASANA
BOAT POSTURE

BENEFITS: Boat Posture strengthens the hips, back, and abdominals and encourages bandha control.

> **CONTRAINDICATIONS:** DO NOT PRACTICE WHEN PREGNANT.

❶ INHALE: Jump through with both legs straight. As you sit down, lift your legs and spine 45 degrees off the floor. Your toes should be level with the top of your head. Bring your arms parallel to the floor and to each other, keeping your shoulders and back straight.

> **TIP:** Navasana requires the spine and thighs to be at the correct angle if it is to be held safely. To set this angle, sit with your knees bent, hold your kneecaps, and lean back with your arms straight. Lift your sternum and lower back and open your shoulders, then take your feet off the floor and release your hands so that your palms face in to your knees. Straighten your legs as much as possible while keeping your back straight.

❷ EXHALE: Hold for 5 breaths.

❸ INHALE: Cross your legs, place your hands on the floor, and lift.

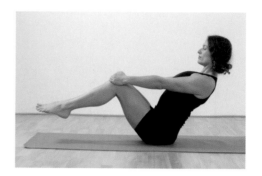

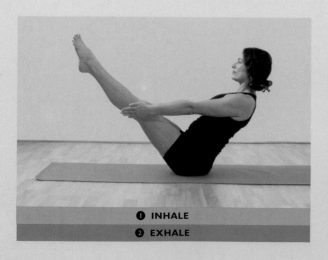

❶ INHALE
❷ EXHALE

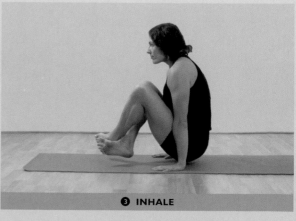

❸ INHALE

❹ EXHALE: Sit down, bringing your arms parallel to the floor.

❺ INHALE: Come back up into Navasana, and repeat 5 times in total, finishing with a Vinyasa.

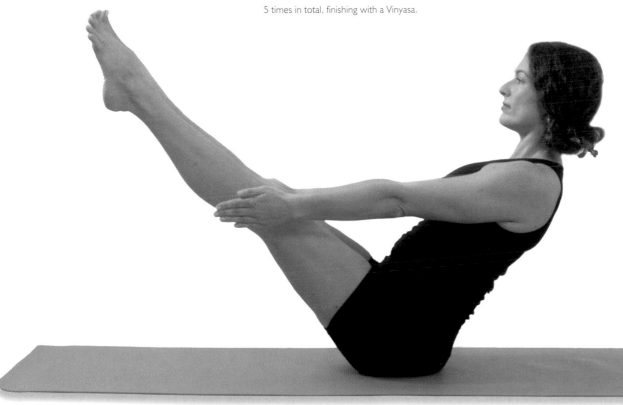

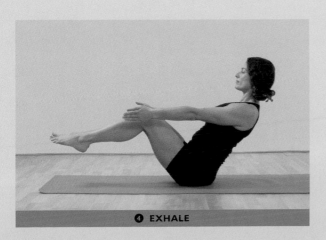

❹ EXHALE

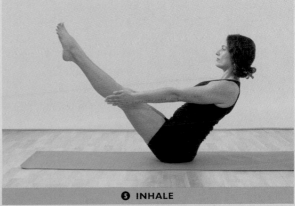

❺ INHALE

THE PRIMARY SERIES

BHUJAPIDASANA
SHOULDER PRESS

BENEFITS: Shoulder Press strengthens the arms and shoulders and increases flexibility in the hips and lower back.

CONTRAINDICATIONS: START WORKING ON THIS POSTURE ONLY AFTER MASTERING THE POSTURES UP TO NAVASANA, OR UNDER THE SUPERVISION OF A TEACHER. DO NOT PRACTICE WHEN PREGNANT.

TIPS: You may need to work on this posture more slowly, starting by jumping your feet either side of your hands first, and then walking them in to position. Lowering your head to the floor can be scary, and most people start by just bringing the forehead down first.

❶ INHALE: Jump your legs around your arms, crossing your right foot over the left.

❷ EXHALE: Lean forward and draw your crossed feet through your arms to bring your head—ideally, the chin—to the floor in front of your hands. Look at your nose. **Hold for 5 breaths.**

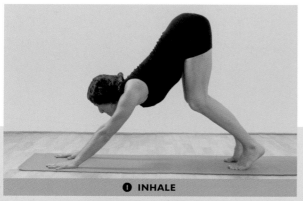

❶ INHALE

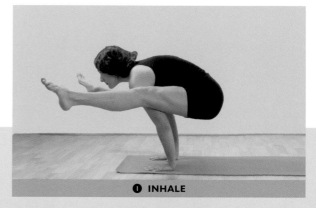

❶ INHALE

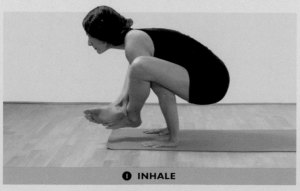

❶ INHALE

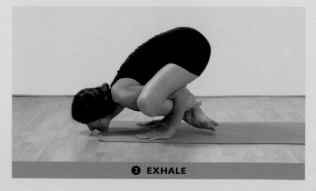

❷ EXHALE

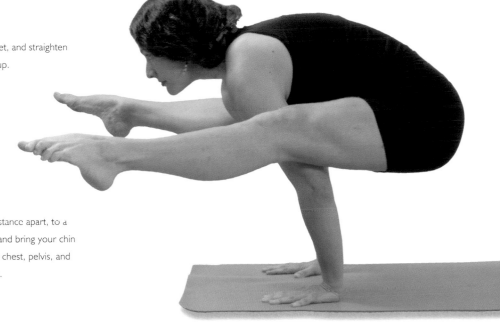

❸ INHALE: Lift up, release your feet, and straighten your arms and legs to balance. Look up.

❹ EXHALE: Bring your feet back so your knees rest on your upper arms.

❺ INHALE: Lift and straighten your arms.

❻ EXHALE: Jump back, feet hip distance apart, to a push-up position. Bend your elbows and bring your chin one inch from the floor, keeping your chest, pelvis, and knees off the floor. Look at your nose.

❼ Finish your Vinyasa as usual.

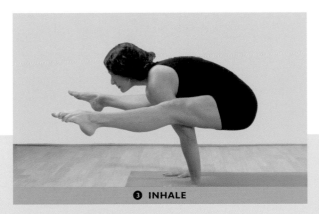

❸ INHALE

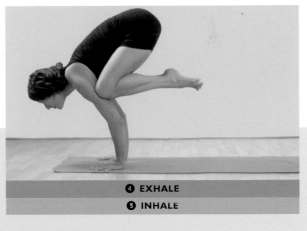

❹ EXHALE
❺ INHALE

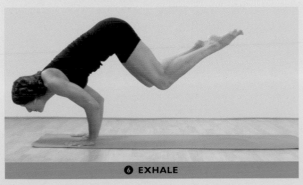

❻ EXHALE

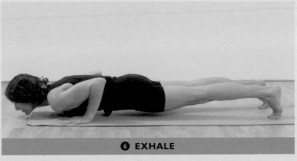

❻ EXHALE

KURMASANA
THE TORTOISE

BENEFITS: Kurmasana continues to open the hips and lower back and broadens the chest, helping to develop the heart and lungs. The mind draws inward and becomes calm.

CONTRAINDICATIONS: DO NOT PRACTICE WHEN PREGNANT.

❶ INHALE: Jump from Downward Dog to land with your feet around your arms. Your knees should be as high on your shoulders as possible. Bend your arms and lower your buttocks to the floor, then extend your arms out to the sides.

TIP: Before pushing your heels forward, make sure they are no more than two feet apart. When working in this posture, keep your legs high up on your arms and close to your sides. Once you are down, push back with your shoulders, open your chest, and lift your head.

❷ EXHALE: Push your heels forward to straighten your legs. Take your heels off the ground and keep the feet flexed and vertical. Look up at the Third Eye. **Hold for 5 breaths.**

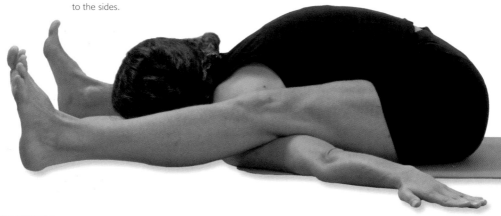

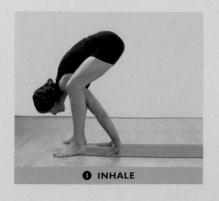

❶ INHALE

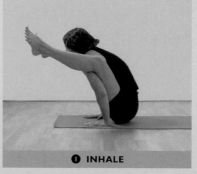

❶ INHALE

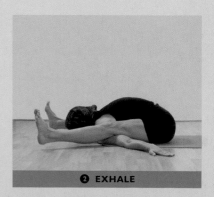

❷ EXHALE

SUPTA KURMASANA
SLEEPING TORTOISE

CONTRAINDICATIONS: DO NOT ATTEMPT THIS POSTURE UNLESS YOU CAN DO KURMASANA.

❶ INHALE: Bend your knees to bring your legs behind your head. Cross your right foot over your left. Move your arms around behind your back and clasp your hands.

> **TIP:** Take extra time to work on the stages, working first with your legs and then with your arms or vice versa. You may need adjusting by a teacher in this position.

❷ EXHALE: Push your shoulders and head back. Look up at the Third Eye. **Hold for 5 breaths.**

❸ INHALE: Release your hands and place them on the floor in front of your buttocks. Lift your body up. Lift up, release your feet, and straighten your arms and legs to balance. Look up. Release your feet and bring them back so your knees rest on your upper arms. Lift and straighten your arms.

❹ EXHALE: Jump back, feet hip distance apart, to a push-up position. Bend your elbows and bring your chin one inch from the floor, keeping your chest, pelvis, and knees off the floor. Look at your nose.

❺ Finish your Vinyasa as usual.

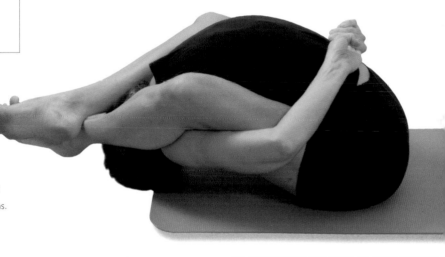

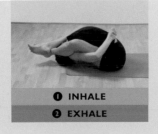
❶ INHALE
❷ EXHALE

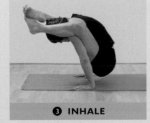
❸ INHALE

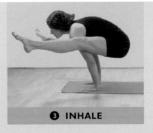
❸ INHALE

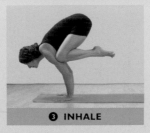
❸ INHALE

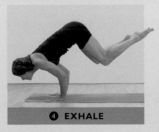
❹ EXHALE

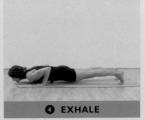
❹ EXHALE

GARBHA PINDASANA
FETUS IN THE WOMB

BENEFITS: This contraction of the abdominal organs, especially the spleen and liver, improves the blood supply. This posture also massages the spine.

> **CONTRAINDICATIONS:** DO NOT PRACTICE THE FULL POSTURE WHEN PREGNANT.

> ### MODIFICATION
> When pregnant, practice Full Lotus on both sides to keep your pelvis evenly open.

❶ INHALE: Jump through with both legs straight, then bring your feet into Full Lotus, right leg first. Lift your knees and, balancing on your sitting bones, (EXHALE:) weave your right hand and arm through the gap between your right calf and thigh and left ankle. Keep your palm face down until you are past your elbow, then bend your arm, palm up. (INHALE:) Repeat on the left side.

> **TIP:** Wearing shorts and a short-sleeved or sleeveless top and using water to lubricate bare arms and legs will enable the arms to slide more easily into place.

❷ EXHALE: Bring your hands to your ears and balance. Look at your nose. **Hold for 5 breaths.**

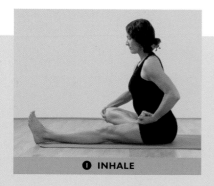

❶ INHALE

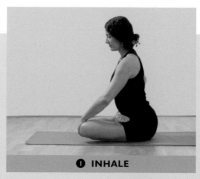

❶ INHALE

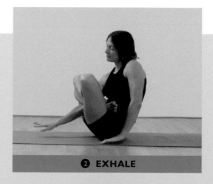

❷ EXHALE

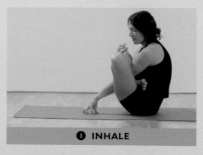

❶ INHALE

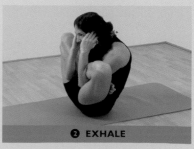

❷ EXHALE

❸ INHALE: Release your hands from your ears. Tuck your head into your hands to curve your spine.

❹ EXHALE: Rock back, rotating clockwise.

❺ INHALE: Rock up.

❻ EXHALE: Rock back and repeat the rocking a total of nine times, continuing to rotate until you are facing forward again.

> **TIP:** Many teachers advise rocking back and up 9 times to symbolize the nine months spent in the womb.

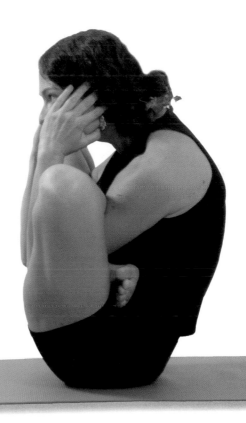

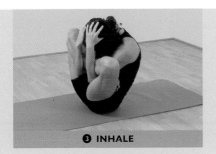

❸ INHALE

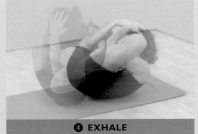

❹ EXHALE

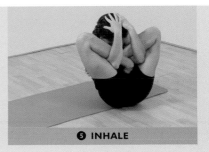

❺ INHALE

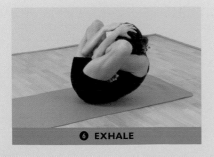

❻ EXHALE

KUKKUTASANA
THE ROOSTER

BENEFITS: This balancing posture strengthens the wrists and abdomen.

CONTRAINDICATIONS: DO NOT PRACTICE WHEN PREGNANT.

❶ INHALE: Rock all the way up from Fetus and release your hands to the floor. Lift your head, open your chest, and balance. Look at your nose. **Hold for 5 breaths.**

TIP: You may need to rock up several times at first to gain enough momentum to balance on your hands.

❷ EXHALE: Sit down and release your arms.

❸ INHALE: Place your hands on the floor and lift.

❹ EXHALE: Swing the lotus through your arms and jump back as part of your Vinyasa.

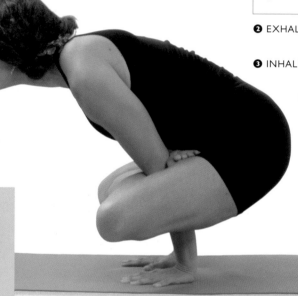

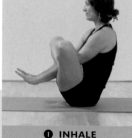

❶ INHALE

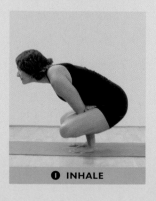

❶ INHALE

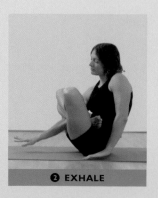

❷ EXHALE

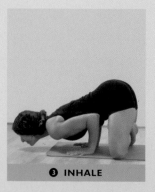

❸ INHALE

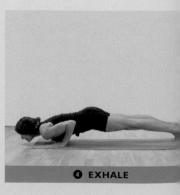

❹ EXHALE

BADDHA KONASANA
COBBLER'S SEAT

BENEFITS: This hip opening pose relieves menstrual problems and strengthens the bladder, and is beneficial during pregnancy.

❶ INHALE: Jump through with straight legs. Bend your legs and bring your heels together toward your groin, knees out to the sides. Hold the top and inside of your feet open like a book, and press your knees to the floor.

❷ EXHALE: Extending through the front of your body, fold at your hips to bring your chin to the floor in front of your feet. Look at your nose. **Hold for 5 breaths.**

> **TIP:** This posture can be extremely challenging. Frequent and painful adjustments by a teacher may be necessary and emotional release is common. Breath control and conscious relaxation of the muscles of the groin are essential. Massaging the hips and quadriceps before working into the posture will help.

❸ INHALE: Look up.

❹ EXHALE: Bring your forehead to your feet. Look at your nose. **Hold for 5 breaths.**

❺ INHALE: Sit up.

❻ EXHALE: Bring your hands to the floor and cross your feet.

❼ INHALE: Do your Vinyasa.

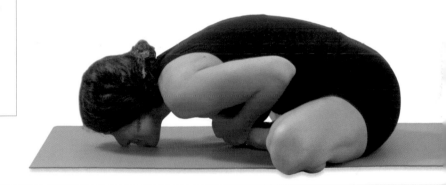

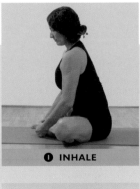

❶ INHALE

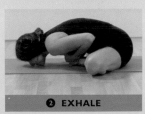

❷ EXHALE

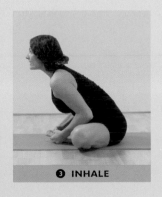

❸ INHALE

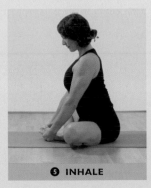

❹ EXHALE

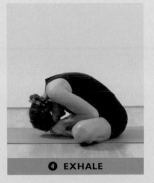

❺ INHALE

UPAVISHTA KONASANA
SEATED ANGLE POSE

BENEFITS: This pose is benefical for menstrual problems and PMS. It also benefits gynecological disorders and is safe during pregnancy if there is no strain. In addition, it stretches the sciatic nerve and the hamstrings.

> **MODIFICATION**
> When pregnant you may want to put your elbows on the floor instead of holding your feet. Do not lift up to balance.

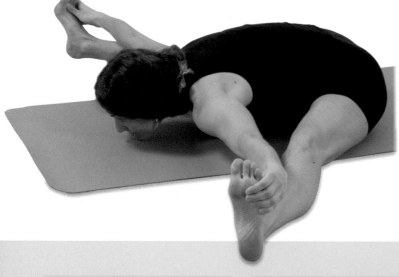

❶ INHALE: Jump through with straight legs. Spread your legs apart at a 90-degree angle. (EXHALE:) Reach down and hold the sides of your feet, thumb below the first and second toe. (INHALE:) Look up, lift your chest, and draw your shoulders back to extend your spine.

❷ EXHALE: Fold at your hips and place your belly, chest, and chin on the floor. Look at your Third Eye. **Hold for 5 breaths.**

❸ INHALE: Lift your legs up to balance on your sitting bones while still holding your feet. Look up. **Hold for 5 breaths.**

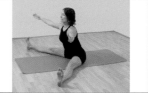
TIP: You may need to let go of your feet to get up.

❹ EXHALE: Bring your hands to the floor and cross your feet.

❺ INHALE: Do your Vinyasa.

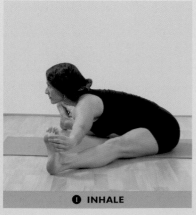
❶ INHALE

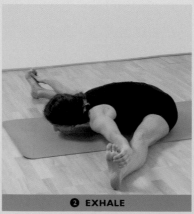
❷ EXHALE

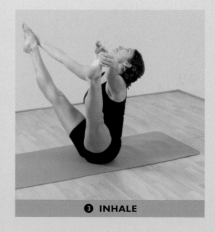
❸ INHALE

SUPTA KONASANA
SUPINE ANGLE POSE

BENEFITS: The spinal massage that is given invigorates the nervous system. The posture requires and encourages bandha control.

> **CONTRAINDICATIONS:** DO NOT PRACTICE WHILE PREGNANT.

TIP: Keep your legs completely straight and draw your toes back throughout the posture. If you bend your knees when rocking up and over, your heels will hit the floor first, and that may hurt. If the posture is held correctly your calves will land first.

❶ INHALE: Jump through with both legs straight.

❷ EXHALE: Lie down.

❸ INHALE: Bring your legs up and over your head, 90 degrees apart.

❹ EXHALE: Put your toes on the floor, and hold your big toes with the first two fingers and thumb of each hand. Lift your sitting bones. Look at your nose. **Hold for 5 breaths.**

❺ INHALE: Roll forward and balance briefly on your buttocks, keeping your arms and legs straight.

❻ EXHALE: Lower your legs, belly, chest, and chin to the floor.

❼ INHALE: Look up.

❽ EXHALE: Release your toes and bring your hands to the floor. Cross your feet.

❾ INHALE: Do your Vinyasa.

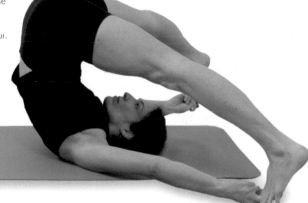

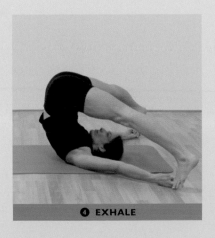

❹ EXHALE

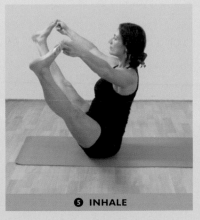

❺ INHALE

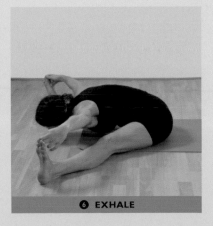

❻ EXHALE

SUPTA PADANGUSTHASANA
SUPINE LEG RAISES

BENEFITS: These Leg Raises help stretch the hamstrings.

❶ INHALE: Jump through with both legs straight.

❷ EXHALE: Lie down.

❸ INHALE: Place your left hand on your left thigh and flex your left foot. Lift your right leg and grasp your big toe with the first two fingers and thumb of your left hand.

❹ EXHALE: Point the toes of both feet and bring your chin to your right knee by drawing your leg down and lifting your upper back off the floor. Look at the toes of your raised leg. **Hold for 5 breaths.**

❺ INHALE: Bring your head to the floor.

❻ EXHALE: Take your leg out to the side, bringing your foot to the floor but keeping your buttocks grounded. Look left. **Hold for 5 breaths.**

❼ INHALE: Bring your head and leg back up to center, still holding your toe.

❽ EXHALE: Draw your chin to your knee.

❾ INHALE: Release your foot and bring your leg to vertical as your head comes down again.

❿ EXHALE: Bring your leg straight down to the floor.

⓫ Repeat on the left side.

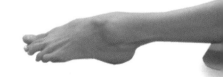

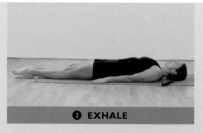

❷ EXHALE

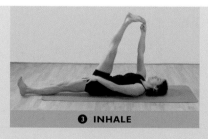

❸ INHALE

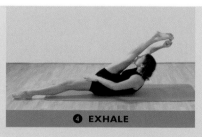

❹ EXHALE

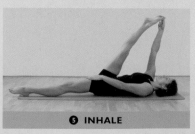

❺ INHALE

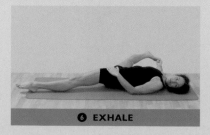

❻ EXHALE

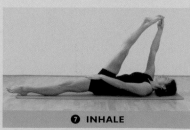

❼ INHALE

TIP: It is common practice to give the legs an intense stretch at the end of this posture. To do so, as you inhale, lift your right leg straight up and grasp your ankle or foot with both hands, or hold your right wrist with your left hand around your foot. As you exhale, draw your leg slightly to the side and down to the floor outside your right ear. Hold for 5 breaths, then inhale to release your foot and exhale to bring it down. Repeat on the left side.

⓬ INHALE: With your arms at your sides, lift your legs and buttocks, directing your toes toward the back of the room. Place your hands either side of your head and press to roll over your head as you push your legs backward.

⓭ EXHALE: Land with your feet hip distance apart in a push-up position. Bend your elbows and bring your chin 1 inch from the floor, keeping your chest, pelvis, and knees off the floor. Look at your nose.

⓮ Complete your Vinyasa.

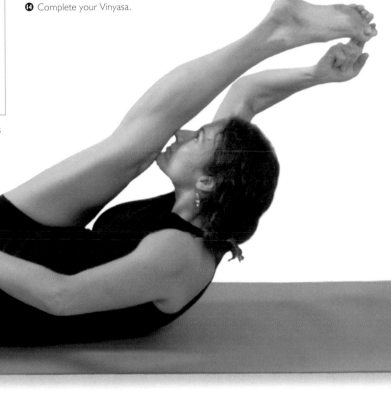

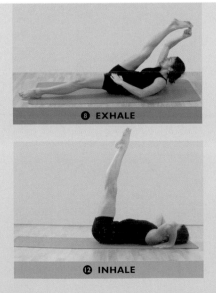

❽ EXHALE

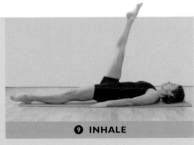

❾ INHALE

❿ EXHALE

⓬ INHALE

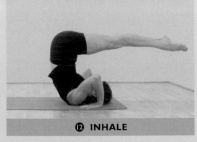

⓬ INHALE

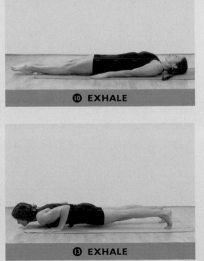

⓭ EXHALE

THE PRIMARY SERIES

UBHAYA PADANGUSTHASANA
BOUND TOE SEATED BALANCE

BENEFITS: This balancing pose purifies and strengthens the abdomen, anus, and genitals.

> **CONTRAINDICATIONS:** DO NOT PRACTICE WHEN PREGNANT.

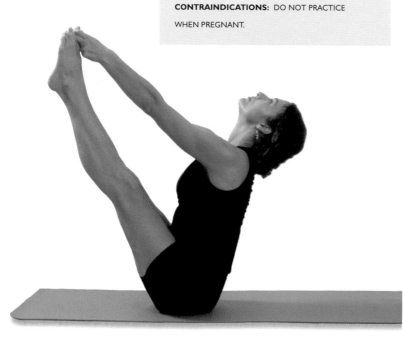

❶ INHALE: Jump through with both legs straight.

❷ EXHALE: Lie down.

❸ (INHALE:) Lift straight legs up and on to the floor behind your head. Keep your legs together.

❹ (EXHALE:) Hold your big toes with the first two fingers and thumb of each hand. Lift your sitting bones and look at your nose. Prepare to rock up by leaning back into your head and using bandha control.

❺ INHALE: Roll up using the strength in your abdomen.

❻ EXHALE: Lean back, pointing your toes to increase the lift. Lift your chest and allow your head to come back. Look at your Third Eye. **Hold for 5 breaths.**

❼ EXHALE: Bring your hands to the floor and cross your feet.

❽ INHALE: Do your Vinyasa.

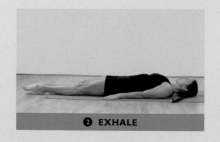

❷ EXHALE

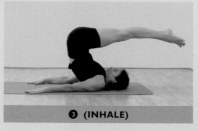

❸ (INHALE)

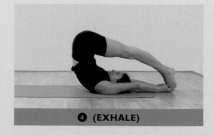

❹ (EXHALE)

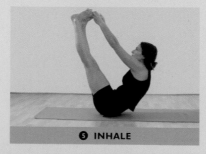

❺ INHALE

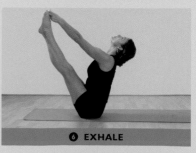

❻ EXHALE

URDHVA MUKHA PASCHIMOTTANASANA
FACE UP FORWARD BEND

BENEFITS: This Forward Bend purifies and strengthens the abdomen, anus, and genitals and develops poise and balance.

> **CONTRAINDICATIONS:** DO NOT PRACTICE WHEN PREGNANT.

❶ **INHALE:** Jump through with both legs straight.

❷ **EXHALE:** Lie down.

❸ **(INHALE:)** Lift straight legs up and over on to the floor behind your head. Keep your legs together.

❹ **(EXHALE:)** Grasp your heels with both hands, lift your sitting bones, and look at your nose. Prepare to rock up by leaning back into your head and using bandha control.

❺ **INHALE:** Roll up using the strength in your abdomen. Lift your head, extend your spine, and keep your legs straight.

❻ **EXHALE:** Take your chin to your shins. Look at your feet. **Hold for 5 breaths.**

❼ **INHALE:** Lean back, keeping your legs and spine straight.

❽ **EXHALE.** Bring your hands to the floor and cross your feet.

❾ **INHALE:** Do your Vinyasa.

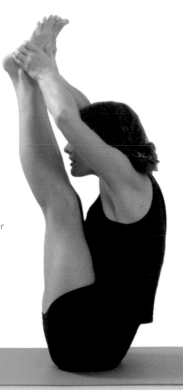

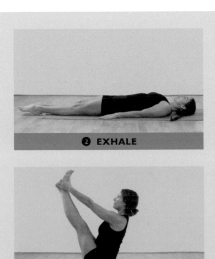
❷ EXHALE

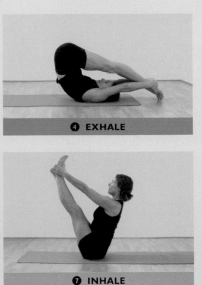
❸ INHALE

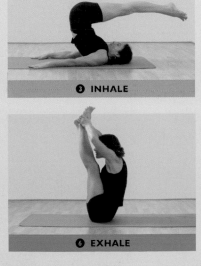
❹ EXHALE

❺ INHALE

❻ EXHALE

❼ INHALE

SETU BANDHASANA
BOUND BRIDGE

BENEFITS: A good preparation for back bending, this posture strengthens the neck and back muscles and tones the reproductive system.

CONTRAINDICATIONS: DO NOT PERFORM THIS POSE IF YOU SUFFER FROM NECK INJURIES.

❶ **INHALE:** Jump through with both legs straight.

MODIFICATION
When pregnant, replace with modified back bends, keeping your shoulders on the floor, arms by your sides, and lifting only your pelvis.

❷ **EXHALE:** Lie down. Bring your heels together around two and one-half hand lengths from your groin, toes pointing out. Lift on to your elbows to arch your back and come on to the top of your head. Cross your arms over your chest.

❸ **INHALE:** Press through your feet and straighten your legs, bringing your buttocks off the mat, and roll over your head on to your hairline. Look at your nose. Hold for 5 breaths.

TIP: Work into the posture carefully. If you prefer, leave your hands palm down on the floor by your sides and use them to balance. Do not place the hands on either side of your head, as this will prevent your neck muscles from developing.

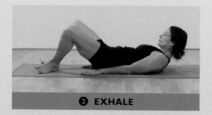

❷ EXHALE

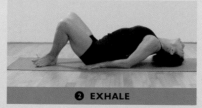

❷ EXHALE

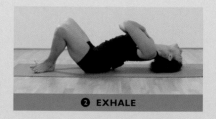

❷ EXHALE

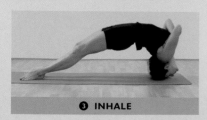

❸ INHALE

❹ EXHALE: Bend your knees and lower to the floor, release your head, and straighten your legs.

❺ INHALE: With your arms by your head, lift your legs and buttocks over your head, bringing your toes down towards the floor. Place your hands either side of your head and press to roll over your head as you push your legs backward with your toes on the floor.

❻ EXHALE: Land with your feet hip distance apart in a push-up position. Bend your elbows and bring your chin one inch from the floor, keeping your chest, pelvis, and knees off the floor. Look at your nose.

❼ Complete your Vinyasa.

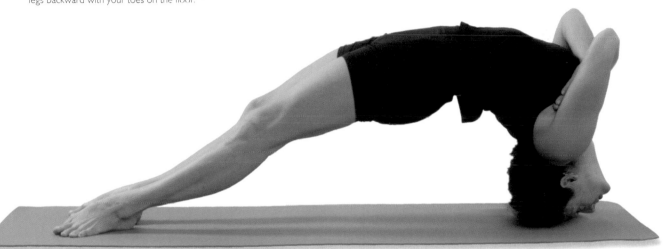

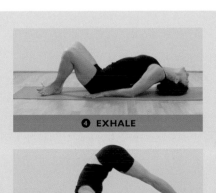

❹ EXHALE

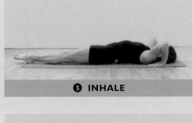

❺ INHALE

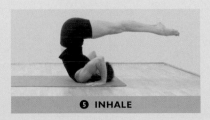

❺ INHALE

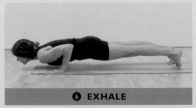

❺ INHALE

❻ EXHALE

URDHVA DHANURASANA
FACE UP BOW

BENEFITS: This serves as an energizer and anti-depressant. It strengthens the arms and shoulders, increases the flexibility of the spine and shoulders, and stretches the pectoral area to improve circulation and tone the muscles supporting the breasts. It also helps regulate the menstrual cycle and eases symptoms of menopause.

❶ **INHALE:** Jump through with both legs straight.

❷ **EXHALE:** Lie down. Bend your legs and place your feet just forward of the outside of your hips, feet parallel. Put your hands either side of your head, slightly wider than shoulder distance apart, fingers pointing in.

❸ **INHALE:** Press evenly with your hands and feet to lift up into a back bend. Look at your nose. **Hold for 5 breaths.**

❹ **EXHALE:** Lower yourself on to the top of your head. Bring your hands and feet a bit closer together. Repeat 3 times in total.

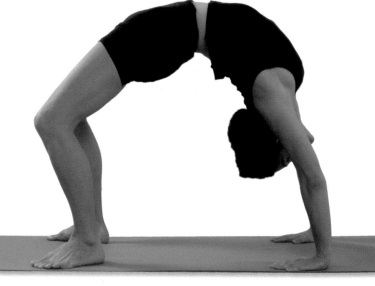

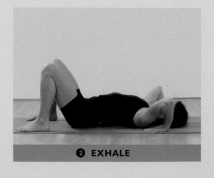
❷ EXHALE

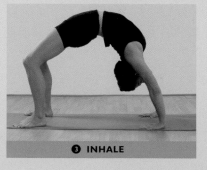
❸ INHALE

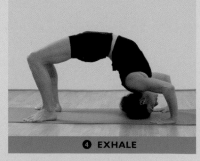
❹ EXHALE

MODIFICATION

With knees bent as for full back bend, keep your arms by your sides, palms down, and lift your pelvis off the floor.

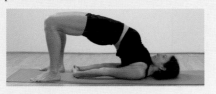

❺ INHALE: Sit up straight. Lean forward and lock your hands around your feet, holding your wrist if possible. Lengthen your torso.

❻ EXHALE: Fold forward. Look toward your feet. **Hold for 10 breaths.**

❼ INHALE: Look up, maintaining your grip.

❽ EXHALE: Bring your hands to the floor and cross your feet.

❾ INHALE: Do your Vinyasa.

CONTRAINDICATIONS: MAY NOT BE SUITABLE FOR THOSE WITH HEART PROBLEMS, HIGH BLOOD PRESSURE, BAD BACKS, INJURED KNEES, OR DURING MENSTRUATION. PRACTICE A MODIFIED BACK BEND WHEN PREGNANT, KEEPING SHOULDERS ON THE FLOOR, ARMS BY YOUR SIDES, AND ONLY LIFTING THE PELVIS.

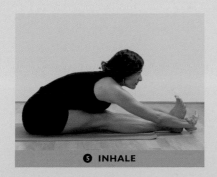

❺ INHALE

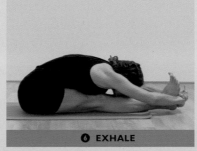

❻ EXHALE

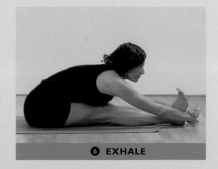

❻ EXHALE

THE FINISHING SEQUENCE

The inverted postures of the finishing sequence revitalize the system, activate sluggish internal organs, improve circulation and the immune system, tone the glandular system, and aid concentration and sleep. All inverted postures help in normalizing the menstrual cycle when part of the regular practice. The mantra below can be recited after the Breathing Sequence at the end of the practice.

Mangala Mantra

Om
Swasti- Praja Bhyaha, pari pala yantam
Nya- yena Margena mahi mahishaha
Go bramanebhyaha- shubhamastu- nityam
Lokaa Samastha Sukhino bhavantu
Om

Om
May we recognize the divine in our abundance
May our leaders rule the world with law and justice
May we always have the right to worship and study freely
And may the people of the whole world be happy and prosperous
Om

SALAMBA SARVANGASANA
SHOULDER STAND

BENEFITS: Shoulder Stand strengthens the nervous system and stimulates the thyroid and parathyroid glands, regulating the metabolism. It tones the reproductive system, helps with prolapsed uterus, and relieves symptoms of menopause.

> **CONTRAINDICATIONS:** Not suitable for those with heart problems, high blood pressure, detached retina, ear infections, or during menstruation.

MODIFICATION

When pregnant, practice with care. You may prefer to lie with your legs resting up the wall instead of doing full Shoulder Stand. Avoid the variations.

❶ INHALE: Jump through with both legs straight.

❷ EXHALE: Lie down.

❸ INHALE: Lift straight legs up and over on to the floor behind your head. Keep your legs together. Place your hands on to your back as close to the shoulder blades as possible and lift your legs straight up. If you press your shoulders and head down you should be able to release any pressure in your neck. Look at your nose. **Hold for 30 breaths.**

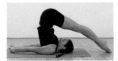

Tip: Lace your fingers and extend your arms straight out behind your back to bring your elbows closer together, then lift higher on to your shoulders.

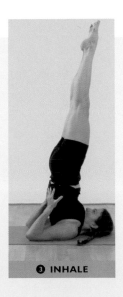

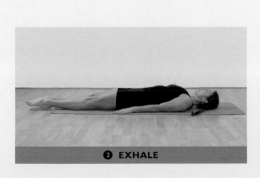

❷ EXHALE

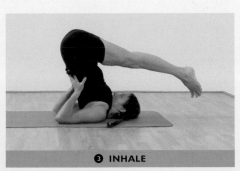

❸ INHALE

❸ INHALE

HALASANA
PLOW

❶ EXHALE: From Shoulder Stand, lower your legs over your head to the floor. Keep your toes pointed. Lace your fingers and extend your arms so your hands touch the ground. Look at your nose. **Hold for 15 breaths.**

❷ INHALE: Prepare for the next posture.

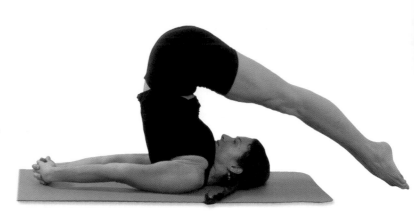

KARNAPIDASANA
EAR SQUEEZE

BENEFITS: The body and mind relax.

❶ EXHALE: Bend your legs, keeping your feet together, and bring your knees to the floor on either side of your head. Squeeze your ears with your knees and press your knees to the floor. Look at your nose. **Hold for 10 breaths.**

❷ INHALE: Bring your hands up to support your back and lift your legs back up into Shoulder Stand.

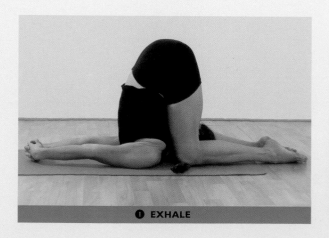

❶ EXHALE

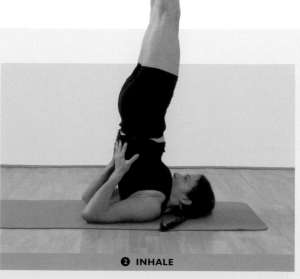

❷ INHALE

URDHVA PADMASANA
FACE UP LOTUS

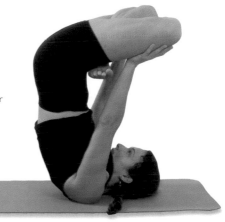

BENEFITS: This provides a strong upward stretch.

❶ EXHALE: Bring your legs into Lotus position, right leg first.

❷ INHALE: Rest your knees on your hands and straighten your arms to lift your knees. Look at your nose. **Hold for 5 breaths.**

PINDASANA
FETUS

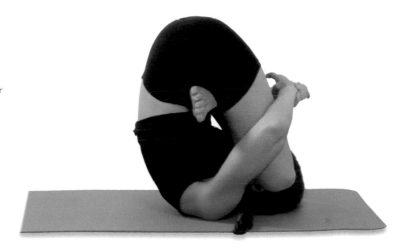

❶ EXHALE: Lower your knees to your ears, wrap your arms around your legs, and clasp your hands. Look at your nose. **Hold for 5 breaths.**

❷ INHALE: Release your arms to the floor, palms down for support.

❸ EXHALE: Roll down with control, bringing your buttocks to the floor and maintaining the Lotus.

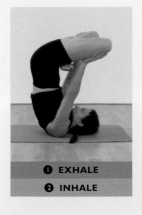

❶ EXHALE
❷ INHALE

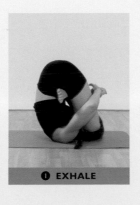

❶ EXHALE

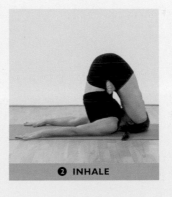

❷ INHALE

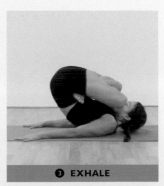

❸ EXHALE

MATSAYASANA
FISH

BENEFITS: Regular practice of Fish will strengthen
a prolapsed uterus. The pose stretches the pectoral
area to improve circulation and tone the muscles
supporting the breasts.

❶ INHALE: Lift on to your elbows to bring your knees
down from Fetus. Arch your back and lower your head
to the floor.

❷ EXHALE: Hold your feet and straighten your arms.
Look at your Third Eye. **Hold for 5 breaths.**

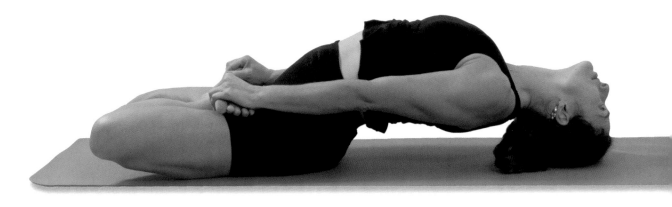

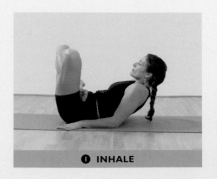

❶ INHALE

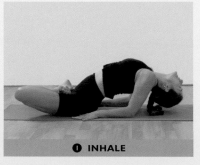

❶ INHALE

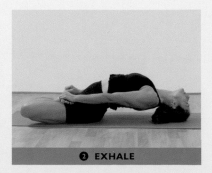

❷ EXHALE

UTTANAPADASANA
LEG EXTENSION

❶ INHALE: Release your legs from Lotus and bring them straight up to 45 degrees from the floor. Bring your hands into prayer position and straighten your arms so your straight fingers point toward your toes. Look at your nose. **Hold for 5 breaths.**

❷ EXHALE: Bring your hands to the floor on either side of your head and release your neck, keeping your legs off the ground.

❸ INHALE: Lift your legs up and over your head. As your buttocks come off the ground, press to roll over your head as you push your legs back.

❹ EXHALE: Land with your feet hip distance apart in a push-up position. Bend your elbows and bring your chin two inches from the floor, keeping your chest, pelvis, and knees off the floor. Look at your nose.

❺ INHALE: Upward Dog.

❻ EXHALE: Downward Dog.

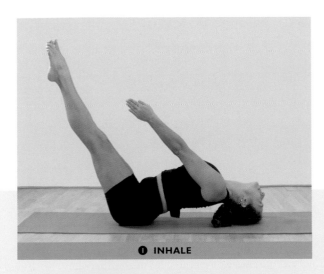

❶ INHALE

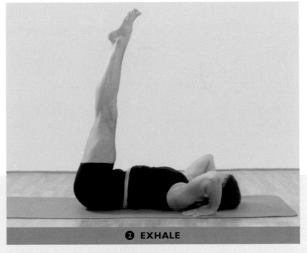

❷ EXHALE

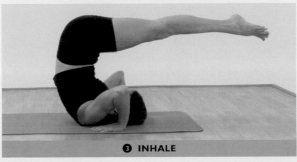

❸ INHALE

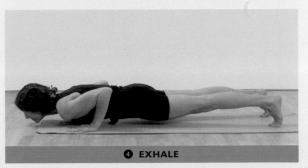

❹ EXHALE

SIRSASANA
HEAD STAND AND VARIATIONS

BENEFITS: Head Stand stimulates the brain and activates the pituitary gland. It also relieves symptoms of menopause.

MODIFICATION

As with Shoulder Stand, during the last three months of pregnancy practice with care and against a wall for support or not at all.

---

❶ INHALE: From Downward Dog, kneel and set the base of the Head Stand. Measure the correct elbow distance by holding your elbows with opposite hands and placing them in front of your knees. Release your elbows and lace your hands.

❷ EXHALE: Place the top of your head between your wrists so the back of your head is supported by the base of your thumbs. Straighten your legs and lift your buttocks.

❸ INHALE: Lift up into Head Stand using your hips as a counterbalance. Look at your nose. **Hold for 25 breaths.**

❹ EXHALE: Lower your legs to 90 degrees. Look at your nose. **Hold for 10 breaths.**

❺ INHALE: Raise your legs back to full Head Stand.

❻ EXHALE: Maintain balance.

❼ INHALE: Push through your arms to lift your head up and off the floor. Flex your feet. Look toward your toes. **Hold for 10 breaths.**

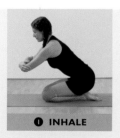

❶ INHALE

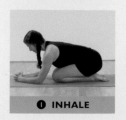

❶ INHALE

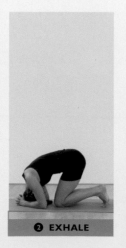

❷ EXHALE

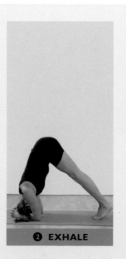

❷ EXHALE

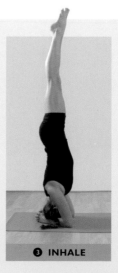

❸ INHALE

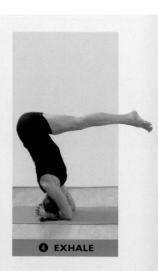

❹ EXHALE

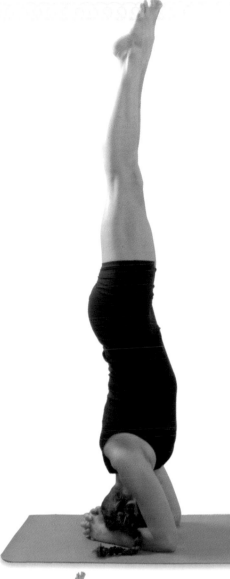

❽ EXHALE: Move back into Head Stand.

❾ INHALE: Prepare to lower.

❿ EXHALE: Bring your legs down straight until your feet reach the floor. Kneel and tuck your chin in so the top of your head rests in front of your feet. Arms come down either side of your legs. **Relax for 25 breaths.**

⓫ INHALE: Do your Vinyasa.

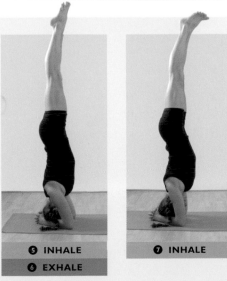
❺ INHALE
❻ EXHALE

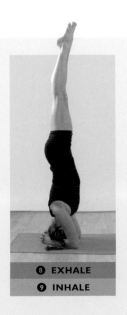
❼ INHALE

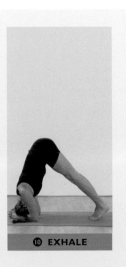
❽ EXHALE
❾ INHALE

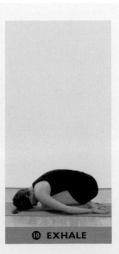
❿ EXHALE

❿ EXHALE

THE BREATHING SEQUENCE

BADDHA PADMASANA
BOUND LOTUS

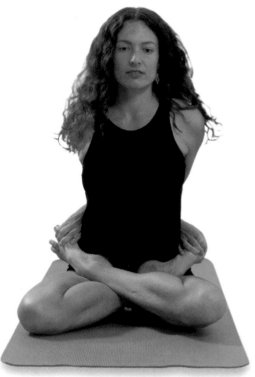

❶ INHALE: Jump through with both legs straight, then bring feet into Full Lotus, right leg first. Bring your left arm behind your back to clasp your left toes, then bring your right arm behind your back to clasp your right toes.

❷ EXHALE: Fold forward, extending your chin to the floor in front of your feet. Look at your Third Eye. **Hold for 10 breaths.**

> **MODIFICATION**
> When pregnant do not fold forward.

❸ INHALE: Sit up and release your hands.

❹ EXHALE: Bring your index finger and thumb together and rest the back of your wrists on your knees. Practice bandha control. Look at your nose. **Hold for 20 breaths.**

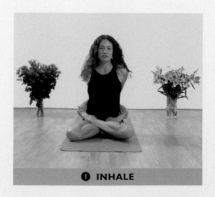

❶ INHALE

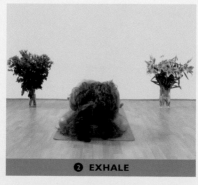

❷ EXHALE

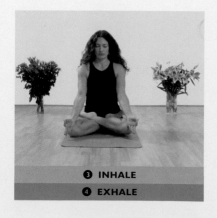

❸ INHALE
❹ EXHALE

UTH PLUTHI
BALANCE

❶ **INHALE:** Bring your hands to the floor slightly forward of your hips while lifting your knees. Lift your body off the mat. Look at your nose. **Hold for 10 breaths.**

❷ **EXHALE:** Sit down. Bring your hands into prayer position. Take as long as you need for prayer, affirmation, or the Mangala Mantra (see page 96).

❸ **INHALE:** Bring your attention back to your practice.

❹ **EXHALE:** Place your hands on the floor.

❺ **INHALE:** Lift your body.

❻ **EXHALE:** Swing the Lotus through your arms and jump back for your final Vinyasa.

RELAXATION

BENEFITS: During relaxation the body heals most effectively and the mind processes what has been learned during the practice. Relaxation can be helpful for PMS, menopausal symptoms, and during menstruation

❶ **INHALE:** Jump through with both legs straight.

❷ **EXHALE:** Lie down on your back with your legs wider than hip distance and your arms out to the sides. Relax for at least 10 minutes, releasing any tension in your body and face, softening the breath and allowing the mind to wander.

> **MODIFICATION**
> While pregnant relax lying on the left side and supported by pillows.

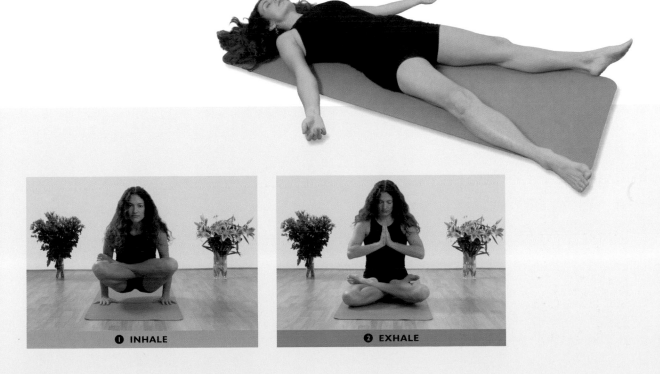

❶ INHALE   ❷ EXHALE

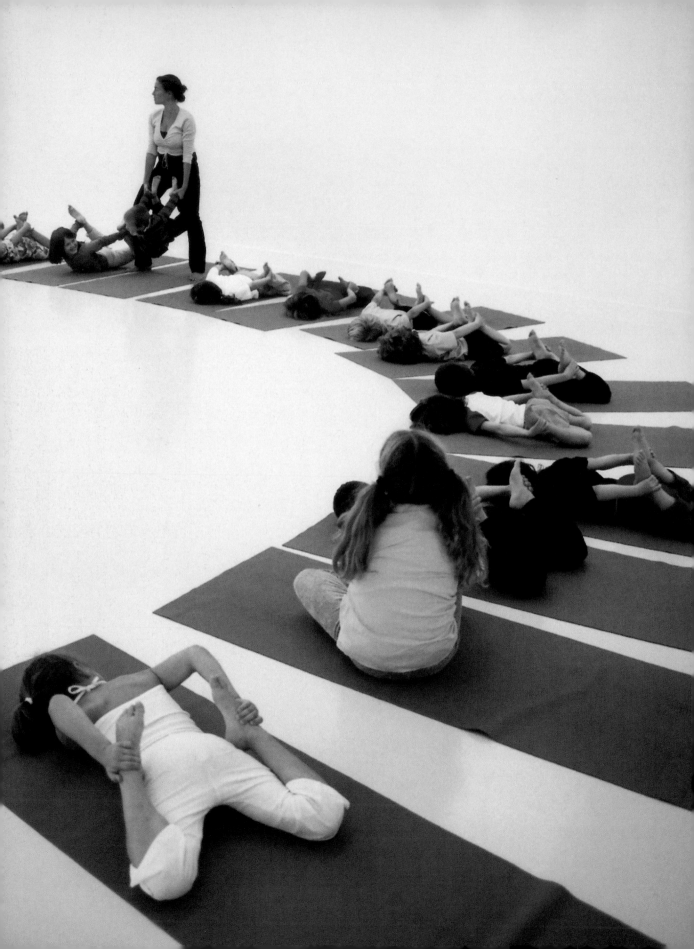

CHAPTER THREE

ASHTANGA AND THE CYCLES OF LIFE

Life is a cycle and as one phase passes another is entered.

Yoga is a path that honors all life's stages. At the heart

of transition is birth and death as we let go of one stage

and receive another. A lifetime of experience is etched

on our bodies and faces. The more flexible and strong

we are, the easier life is. There are healing benefits from

developing a yoga practice that mean we can enjoy yoga

at any level, at any time of our lives. We can start now

and immediately tap into the universal current.

All it takes is the willingness to get on the mat.

THE CYCLES OF LIFE

You need a very long time, and this without having the least result, never getting discouraged and continuing your effort, absolutely regularly, moreover, as though you were quite disinterested about the result. You do the work because you do it. And then, suddenly, one day, it bursts and you see before you the full result of your work.
(The Mother, Sri Aurobindo, Health and Healing in Yoga)

Ashtanga is a series of asanas that heals the body. The Primary Series is the foundation of the practice and the asanas are a way of stimulating and detoxifying the internal organs and developing a strong and healthy body. In addition, the experience of physically opening the body will clear emotional blocks—often held as tension in the body-and free the heart.

Just as Ashtanga is a sequence, so too are the stages of life. Whatever is happening to us on a personal level may be reflected back during the practice.

LUCY AND JOHN SCOTT, U.K.-BASED ASHTANGA TEACHERS. JOHN IS CERTIFIED BY GURUJI AND IS ONE OF THE MOST ADVANCED TEACHERS IN THE WORLD. LUCY IS "BLESSED" BY GURUJI.

Conversely, by listening to our bodies as we move with the asanas we can learn more about ourselves. We can note what an asana brings up for us in terms of thoughts and emotions, and determine how it reflects our thinking in the world.

Asanas are in themselves empty of meaning; difficulty or ease while practicing is a personal experience that varies depending on body type, temperament and for each individual on a daily basis.

There is no age limit to beginning the practice of Ashtanga yoga, although both pace and progression should be slower as we get older. Ashtanga improves the quality of life and brings a certain harmony to the spirit at any age. Many older women find the symptoms of menopause decrease with practice. As The Mother says, "At the end of the sequence you see the full result of your work". Begin Ashtanga practice as soon as possible; progress when you can: this practice is for life.

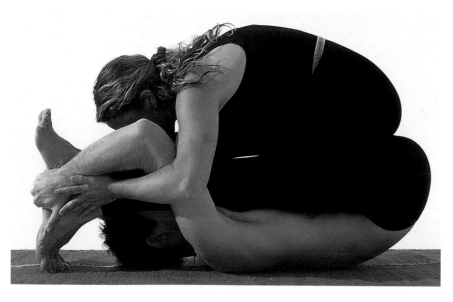

PERSONAL ACCOUNT: LUCY SCOTT

Lucy Scott, an Ashtanga teacher based in England, explains her relationship to her yoga practice:

The practice [of Ashtanga] is a great many things to me. My greatest struggle has been to attend my mat each day. I have on many occasions simply failed to turn up.

I experience my most uplifting and most downhearted practices when alone. Ultimately it is in this state of aloneness that I have the greatest sense of yoga or "yoking"— a union with the divine energy that courses through my veins and the veins of all sentient beings. When I am alone with my breath and that divine energy, I have the greatest chance to glimpse a stillness and a peace that I believe resides in each and every one of us. Each day I have the chance to enter the stillness and dwell in that place but initially and often it eludes me and is overshadowed by all the talk of my busy mind. Nonetheless, as I practice I find that alongside the chattering of my mind there is a growing sense of a quieter state of being becoming available to me. If only for the duration of the practice itself, I am able to move beyond my mental and emotional states and access a sort of neutral. This is the greatest gift for me, to transcend the things I am attached to—if only for a short while—and come to this neutral—this stillness—in me.

I was introduced to the practice of Ashtanga Vinyasa yoga by Derek Ireland and Radha Warrell, who were giving workshops at Danceworks in London. I was taught a little more by a bodywork teacher friend of mine, Ken Eyerman, who had been a student of Derek's for some time. Before the end of 1993, I headed off to India for a journey that was to change the entire course of my life.

Ken Eyerman had told me about a teacher called John Scott who was teaching a workshop in Kovalam, South India. I had been intending to learn an additonal massage technique called *Chavutti Thirimal*, the teacher of which was also based in South India, in Trivandrum. I met John Scott, whose workshop was full, but who kindly invited me and my friend to join him and Gwendoline Hunt in their afternoon practice. John and I then became as we are today—together.

John encouraged me to go to Mysore and work with Guruji and I did. It was there that things began to happen to me. I felt that Guruji could see all of my most vulnerable facets and, in fact, he spoke many poignant and true words to me—although they felt a little painful at the time.

I spent a total of four months with Guruji and my practice became an important part of my life. The energy in the room and the intensity of the yoga there began to move many a hidden thing in me—I was feeling as though I was coming undone—in a good way. I was releasing so many things that I no longer needed to carry, facing myself in a way that I hadn't faced myself before. Going to the mat each day was like going to look in the mirror and it remained like that for a long time.

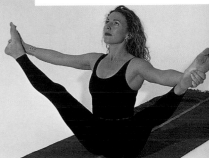

LUCY SCOTT HOLDING UPAVISHTA KONASANA WHILE PRACTICING BROOMADHYA (THIRD EYE DRISHTI).

LYNNE PINETTE ADJUSTS A STUDENT IN ONE OF HER PREGNANCY CLASSES AT THE LIFE CENTRE, LONDON, U.K..

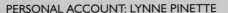

PERSONAL ACCOUNT: LYNNE PINETTE

Lynne Pinette, a sixty-year-old mother, has been practicing Ashtanga and teaching yoga for pregnancy since her mid-fifties:

I personally find it to be a great practice because of the ujjayi breath and bandhas, which produce internal heat, something that disappears with menopause. I daresay my pelvic floor is stronger now than when I was fifty. I have found yoga to be very supportive. It helps relieve psychological symptoms, because one starts to feel good about one's body image and self-esteem, and it gives one hope. I found Ashtanga to have the most dramatic impact—it's not easy, one must work at it—but it is the most effective practice.

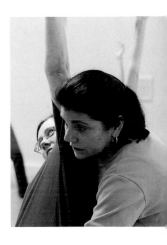

SUN

Ashtanga yoga practice begins with a salute to the sun in a powerful connection to nature and to ancient forms of the divine. The sun has been a central spiritual symbol for people through the ages. Day is the domain of the sun, clearly visible as it rises, peaks, and falls in the sky, providing us with life-giving warmth and sustenance.

Traditionally the Sun Salute would have begun the morning yoga practice as the sun rose in the sky at daybreak. We raise our arms above our heads and expand our hearts in this salute. As our chests open, we take deep breaths and our consciousness becomes filled with the energy of the day. What the sun is to growing plants, it is symbolically to our spirits. Without it we would not be able to live. It gives us energy and is a source of inspiration and joy.

Yoga first developed in India's hot climate and the sun's fierce heat would have prevented practice during the middle of the day. Yogis timed their Sun Salute to coincide with the rising of the sun. The salute to the sun is symbolic of a "beginning" and refers to waking up and becoming aware. Modern lifestyles often leave little time to practice in tune with sunrise, and we often take classes at night or after work. Though we usually practice yoga indoors without reference to the sun's position, it can be a very different experience to do the Sun Salute as the day begins instead of at the end of the day or even at night. Whatever time we do Ashtanga, it always begins with the Sun Salute and reconnects us with the vibrancy of the sun and its symbolic life-sustaining properties.

Cultural differences also impact on the timing of our yoga practice. Global climatic differences mean that we may never have the same experience of yoga from country to country. For those who can do yoga as a morning practice, it makes a good start to the day as it wakes you up and gets your body moving. But early morning yoga may not be an option for those who work or have children and whose circumstances require different timing. Bodies are less stiff later in the day, and this can be a real

THE SUN, AS THE SYMBOL OF ALL LIFE, HAS INSPIRED WORSHIP SINCE THE BEGINNING OF TIME.

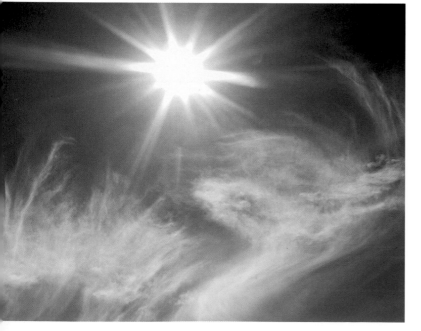

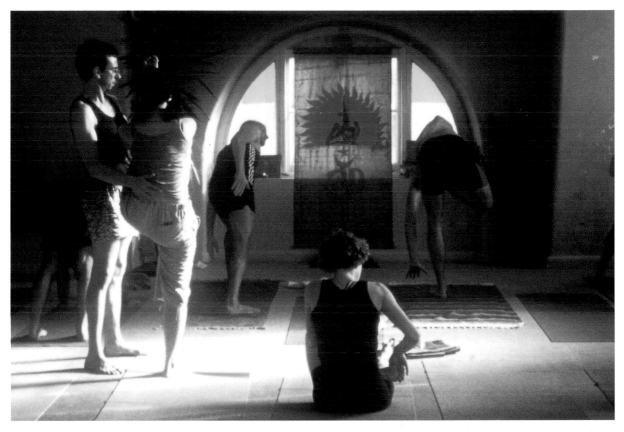

advantage. Bending over first thing in the morning is not as easy as it is in the afternoon. Ultimately, the timing of a regular practice must be flexible enough to work for anyone, and since yoga is about transformation it can be transformative itself in accommodating individual lifestyles.

The Salute to the Sun is a series of asanas designed to move the body into fundamental stretches. The foundation of Ashtanga practice consists of the Sun Salutes A and B, and the key to these asanas is the opening of the heart and chest. In Warrior Pose we take on the courage of a warrior to move affirmatively through life. Courage and the heart are intimately linked, and the heart-opening stretches are designed to launch us confidently into life. Upward Dog and Downward Dog stretch our arms and legs and extend the spine. Our feet in the first asana (Samasthedhi) are rooted to the earth, while our arms reach for the sky. A good foundation mirrors the energy of earth and sky, represented by two of the most ancient symbols of universal divine force, Mother Earth and Father Sky. If our feet are grounded, then our bodies can fly.

THE SUN FILTERS THROUGH DURING A MORNING ASHTANGA CLASS. PRACTICING IN THE MORNING IS A GOOD START TO THE DAY.

MOON

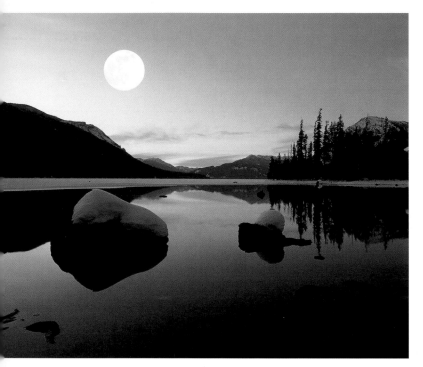

GURUJI STATES THAT
ASHTANGA PRACTICE
SHOULD BE SUSPENDED ON
FULL OR NEW MOON.

The moon's cycle ever-changing from wax to wane and back again is part of the teaching of Ashtanga yoga. For students of Ashtanga it is implicit that they do not practice on the full or new moon. This applies to everyone, both women and men. Guruji says that any injury incurred on these days will take much longer to heal. The underlying reasons for this advice hark back to a lunar system that was understood in ancient India at the time of Patanjali. These two rest days in the month depend on the pull from one kind of energy in the waning phase to another in the waxing phase.

In other ancient spiritual traditions, the moon is a guide for planting crops, for times of healing, and for times of releasing. The moon rules the tides. High tide is at full moon and low tide is at the dark or new moon. For our ancestors, who were much more in touch with nature, the moon cycle was enigmatic and powerful. It was thought that when the moon was full and tides high, human emotion reached peaks. Even the word *lunatic* derives from *Luna*, the Latin name for the goddess of the moon who moved humans in ways that were sometimes excessive. The moon has long been linked symbolically with emotion and there are more accidents and violent outbreaks on, or around, a full moon.

In western symbology, the moon has always been linked with women and the feminine. This is also true in India. It does not mean that men are not also connected to the moon, but the link for women is so strong that many anthropologists believe that women in tribal cultures menstruated at the same time on the dark of the moon. Ovulation would therefore occur on the full of the moon or just before, when the energy was rising.

Without the interruption of modern lighting systems and rushed lifestyles, communities were much more closely connected. Women who rose with the sun and slept under the moon were much more in touch with natural cycles and their menstruation developed a synchronistic rhythm. Women practicing Ashtanga may also find that their menstruation may be in sync with the dark or full of the moon and also with other women in their practice group. This cycle was so important historically that the evolution of words for *moon* are also etymologically connected to *menstruation* and *measurement.* So important was the moon's link to community menstrual and ovulation cycles that spiritual practices developed to channel the different emotional responses of a group. Times of the full and new moon were considered times to stop work and perform other kinds of spiritual practice. At the dark it was time for divination and looking within. At the full it was a time of celebration, sexuality, and group gatherings.

As Ashtanga is a tool for transformation it is possible to conceive of a moon cycle as the time to develop a plan or wish. The practice works in harmony with nature to provide us with a place to work our higher intention. Looking within on the dark of the

moon and meditating upon a transformation that we wish in our lives enables us to move toward it. In meditative states the emotional and spiritual connection to who we really are and to our soul purpose is more direct.

At the end of the finishing sequence in any Ashtanga practice students sit in lotus position for 25 breaths. Though the aim of the sitting is to use the breath to find stillness, it can also be a time of creating positive thoughts that we wish to manifest. In some forms of yoga an intention, called the *Sankalpa*, is a positive affirmation that the individual wishes to manifest. Dedicating healing to another person or to the self, can be sent over a month in the yoga practice. When the body has been cleansed and the mind is clear, the ability to send energy to a problem or a person is magnified. And though this is not the traditional teaching of Ashtanga, there is a space in the practice for possibilities such as these.

... if I feel an affinity with the moon, can I trust the feeling to mean anything, or is it just fantasy? If I feel the pull of the tides on me, if I feel that my period is related to the moon's phases, and arrives with the glory of the full moon and the high tide ... if I feel more restless at the full moon than at other times in the month, if I dream more ... am I to trust these things, or am I "lunatic"? What does it mean, if the moon attracts me, how can I use it in my life?

PENELOPE SHUTTLE AND PETER REDGROVE **THE WISE WOUND**

MENSTRUATION

The roots of the word *menstruation* are derived from the Sanskrit *mati-ha* meaning both "knowing" and "measure." From this comes the Greek *menos*, meaning "spirit," from which evolved words and ideas ranging from heart, soul, and ardor, to madness and mania. From this word also comes *men* or *moon* and the root words for *measurement, cleverness,* and *wisdom.* The evolution of language reflects the dual nature of the moon waxing and waning and of the menstrual cycle's two poles of ovulation and menstruation.

PENELOPE SHUTTLE AND PETER REDGROVE, THE WISE WOUND

Menstruation was considered in ancient cultures to be a time of great internal power and wisdom. It was a time for women to retreat from their daily acitivities and use their energy to do spiritual practices. Early communities perceived giving birth as the single most powerful act a human could perform and it was honored in their spiritual systems. The importance of moon lodges in Native American ritual suggests that the women were in synchronicity when it came to their monthly menstruation. Women would retire to the moon lodge to do magical work together at dark/new moon. This work involved making decisions and performing divination for the community and it was essential to the path of the medicine woman. Menstruation was regarded as one of the most important times for women to commune and receive psychic messages on healing and things that needed attention to be passed on to the whole community.

Full moon coincided with ovulation and was a time of festivity, dancing, feasting, and sexuality. The expansive moon was the visual reminder that groups needed to let off steam and break out of normal routine and celebrate. Many full moon celebrations in various ancient traditions are about love, sex, big ideas, expansion, and demonstrative celebration of the group. Ovulation may be seen as a time of fertility, when women were subconsciously sending out messages to lovers.

The words *menstruation, month,* and *moon* are all related etymologically. They indicate the use of the moon to measure time longer than a day (the role of the sun) and the connection of women's cycles to the moon's cycles. The monthly menstruation cycle played an important part in shaping societies. The month became the structure for activity within a community. In tune with this, Ashtanga makes room within the practice to honor the rest days. Rather than being a time to push ourselves it is a time to dedicate to ourselves.

For women, the exact time of their menstruation marks a time to rest in the Ashtanga practice. Guruji has been known to say that menstrual blood is "unclean," and although this may sound odd, even offensive to some, it has recently been discovered that just before menstruation the liver and kidneys release toxic waste that is removed from the body along with the menstrual blood. This monthly detoxification may provide a partial explanation why women tend to live longer than men.[2]

With regular Ashtanga practice, menstruation should become more efficient—short and heavy, lasting only two or three days. Often this may coincide with the full or new moon and the daily rhythm of the asana practice is barely disturbed. Women vary in their response to menstruation. Some experience little discomfort and want to keep practicing as usual. Others feel heavy or bloated or have painful cramps. Maintaining the practice may feel too difficult. Guruji advises three days off, longer if the bleeding lasts. Inverted postures such as Downward Dog and the finishing asanas must definitely be avoided since the force of gravity works against the menstrual flow.

Ashtanga practice can help with the following problems:

- **Amenorrhea**, when the menses stop completely for a period of time. Geeta Iyengar, daughter of B.K.S. Iyengar, recommends "inversions to increase blood circulation and balance the endocrine system, backbends to tone the liver and twists to massage the internal organs".[3] Increasing the number of breaths during these postures in your daily practice should help.

- **Menstrual cramp**, varying from dull backache to debilitating pain. Gentle yoga postures such as Child's Pose or supported Supine Angle Pose (Supta Baddha Konasana) can help relieve cramp, as can Ujjayi breathing. If cramp is severe and does not improve, seek the advice of a health professional.

- **Premenstrual Syndrome** (PMS), which may be caused by an imbalance of hormones from an inefficient endocrine system and a sluggish liver or malfunctioning pituitary and adrenal glands. By balancing the endocrine system, asanas help release estrogen and progesterone in the correct quantities. A healthy diet and postures that massage the liver will also allow excess hormones to be broken down, passed to the kidneys, and then excreted. Relaxation at the end of the practice eases stress, which helps the hypothalamus regulate the hormones more efficiently.

During the first couple of days of your period look after and within yourself.

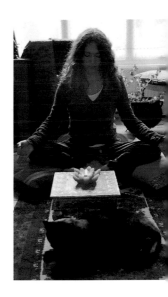

WHEN NOT PRACTICING ASHTANGA DURING MENSTRUATION, TAKE TIME TO REST, REFLECT, AND MEDITATE.

FERTILITY

Many couples are now waiting until they are in their thirties before deciding to have a child. More often now than ever before, women are choosing to wait until they have the security of a stable relationship, a home, and enough money before starting a family. The idea that everything must be in place before deciding may mean that this decision comes at a time in a woman's life when fertility is already on the wane. For many, this delay insures better timing of the event, but for others, who find getting pregnant is not as easy as they imagined, it can be a difficult path of disappointment and frustration. Yoga has become one of the methods that couples have explored in re-evaluating their lifestyles and learning to focus on relaxation and meditation as the first step to achieving pregnancy.

A less stressful lifestyle can help create an environment in which a woman will more easily become pregnant. A hectic lifestyle may result in the failure to conceive, since the over-stressed body cannot prepare for conception to take place. Added to the stress of failure are the feelings of hopelessness when month after month a woman is faced with disappointment. This is the cyclical nature of stress. Often the feeling of inadequacy seems insurmountable, causing women to ask, "Why is this happening to me?" and "What have I done wrong?"

The reasons for infertility may include exposure to environmental toxins, infection-related scarring, hormonal imbalances, thyroid irregularities, smoking, excessive alcohol and drug use, poor diet, and low body fat. Adopting a healthy lifestyle can help. A diet of organic food, high in essential fatty acids and fresh green vegetables, will help cleanse a woman's body. It is also helpful to eliminate coffee and tea, sugar, smoking, and alcohol in order to increase fertility. In addition to dietary changes, a regular yoga practice may help a woman get pregnant since it works to transform both the body and the mind. In a study conducted by the Mind-Body Institute at Harvard University, Herbert Benson, M.D., researcher and

PRACTICING YOGA CAN IMPROVE FERTILITY AND BE A BONDING EXPERIENCE. IT CAN ALSO HELP DURING PREGNANCY. LOUISE WAS DUE TO GIVE BIRTH ON THE DAY THIS PHOTOGRAPH WAS TAKEN.

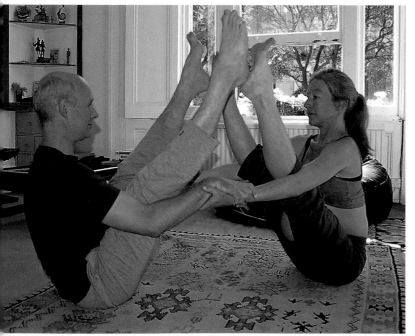

author of *The Relaxation Response*, incorporated stress reduction techniques such as yoga, meditation, and group discussions, in addition to the lifestyle changes already mentioned, and found a 50 percent rise in fertility. Remarkably, these results occurred regardless of the apparent cause of the woman's infertility, including even low sperm count on the part of the male. Another study from Harvard Medical School showed that women who participated in a program of relaxation and yoga were almost three times more likely to get pregnant than women who didn't participate.

Stress is often the result of strong emotions like fear and anger, which cause the body to produce more cortisol and fewer sex hormones. The sympathetic nervous system causes the adrenal glands to release epinephrine into the bloodstream as part of the fight–or–flight reflex to prepare the body for emergency action. Epinephrine also interferes with the body's ability to repair itself and process nourishment, thus increasing the likelihood of infertility. Since epinephrine constricts blood vessels, this constriction may also occur in the uterus. To allow the body to relax and blood to flow freely, there are specific asanas that can stimulate the pelvis and womb. Most hip-opening and pelvic-opening asanas can also help. So too can mild inversion postures that contribute to relaxation.

FINDING BALANCE

Ashtanga is often viewed as a difficult practice and it may be too hard on a system that is already coping with stress. As in any rigorous exercise, the body fat to weight ratio may drop too low and interrupt a woman's menstrual cycle, preserving fertility for a time when the body is ready to nurture a child. However, there is no evidence to show that yoga itself does anything other than make the body healthy. Finding balance is always about getting in touch with your own body and asking the question, "Am I working too hard?" If your practice seems too extreme, eliminate the Vinyasas and work more slowly. Work only half the practice if necessary. Soften and melt into the postures and remember not to become competitive. Be sure to rest as well as practice.

CONTRACEPTIVE ASANAS

Some asanas put a great deal of pressure on the pelvic organs and may act as contraceptives by preventing the embedding of the fertilized egg in the uterine wall. We do not prescribe the use of asanas as a safe method of contraception but include this information as a matter of interest.

The relevant postures are Marichyasana D and Garbha Pindasana, and for those practicing the Second Series, Pasasana, and Yoganidra. Guruji warns women not to perform the abdominal massage Nauli, although his daughter Saraswati thinks that Nauli might encourage menstruation to start when overdue, and has suggested that women experiment to discover the effect on their own bodies when appropriate.

Most beginners are not flexible enough to feel the full effects of these asanas; however, advanced students who are having difficulty becoming pregnant may find it beneficial to ease up on these postures or leave them out altogether.[4]

PREGNANCY

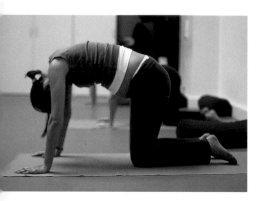

IF ASHTANGA IS TOO HARD FOR BEGINNERS, OTHER YOGA CLASSES ARE OFFERED.

It is recommended that Ashtanga yoga practice should be suspended during the first three months of pregnancy, during which time the placenta is attaching to the uterine wall. During this time, jumping, twisting, and raising the core body temperature are all contraindicated. New students should also avoid inversions altogether, since newcomers may have very little body awareness and might not realize if something goes wrong. Even an experienced practitioner should avoid inversions after the first six months, since inversions alter the flow of energy and may affect the viability of the fetus.

Specific instructions for pregnant women depend on how long they have been practicing yoga and what their bodies are used to in terms of exercise and fitness. A woman with an established practice of several years can resume her practice after the first trimester—with modifications. A woman who is new to the practice, say six months to two years, should enroll in a good prenatal class. The difference for an established practitioner is that her body is used to Ashtanga yoga.

A general rule of thumb is not to start something completely new while you are pregnant. A prenatal yoga class specifically designed for women with minimal experience of yoga would be ideal. Yoga is one of the few practices that can be started during pregnancy, as long as the teacher is trained and very sensitive to the needs of pregnant women. This is especially important during the third trimester, as so many changes will be taking place in the

PERSONAL ACCOUNT: EMMA CATTO

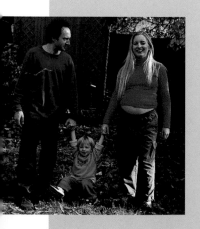

Emma Catto is an Ashtanga teacher, pictured here pregnant with her second child and with her husband, Robin, also an Ashtanga teacher, and their son:

I seem to have a body that feels nauseous for most of the first four months of pregnancy. As someone who is used to feeling strong and fit and using the wonderful tools of yoga to rebalance and retreat, this is incredibly hard. There is no escape; one of the first lessons of parenthood, I suppose. As my body gets more used to pregnancy, it has to be constantly adapted according to the baby's position and my energy and size.

The strengthening and familiarity of certain positions helped me feel more secure in where my body wanted to be [during childbirth], but the core of the birth was in the breathing. Not a particular type of breathing, but being aware of the breath, having the breath as a focus, and using the breath to move, to relax, and to release.

woman's body (for example, the blood volume will increase by 35 to 50 percent), and each asana needs to be taught with great sensitivity.

EVERY WOMAN'S PREGNANCY IS UNIQUE. LISTEN TO YOUR BODY AND DO ONLY WHAT FEELS COMFORTABLE.

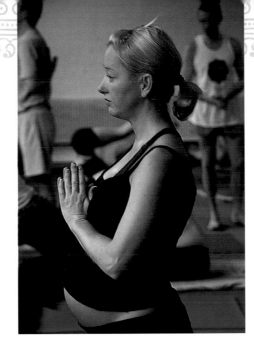

PERSONAL ACCOUNT: LUCY SCOTT

After the third month [of my pregnancy], I stopped going forward in Marichyasana A and B and only did it sitting straight; I didn't want to compress my abdomen at all. I also stopped Marichyasana C and D (all twists). I found replacements by simply twisting away from rather than over the bent leg. I stopped Garbhapindasana after four months and simply rocked along my spine clasping my hands around my knees. I also stopped Kurmasana and Supta Kurmansana. My Vinyasas changed gradually in accordance with what was possible and what felt good. I eventually did Suryanamaskar A and B and all Vinyasas with my legs hip-distance apart or wider as I got larger. I really got into my squats in Suryanamaskar B and developed great power in my legs and bottom. I felt really strong later in my pregnancy. I continued to practice in this first pregnancy right up to the end. I was greatly inhibited, of course, but the breath, the awareness to bandha, and some semblance of asana remained.

When I felt too cumbersome to meet myself on the mat and pregnancy didn't feel like such a gift, I took John's advice: "Just go and stand on your mat—go there, feel where you are today, and just accept it." So I used to stand on my mat, unable to see my feet, and cry.

I've often thought that I would have ended up with a C-section with Fynn's birth had I been in a hospital.

I was adamant that I wanted drug-free home births with both of my children and somehow (foolishly perhaps) never doubted my ability to endure. But the midwives both commented on my breathing and my strength, especially in my legs, and my level of stamina. They thought that it had come from my yoga practice.

Birth is an unfolding process that involves the baby as much as it involves you and, combined with all the complex chemical processes at work, is not something that you can have power or control over. You can simply use techniques to harness its unfolding in the most positive way available to you—or alternatively find a way to disengage from it if it's all too much and opt for an epidural. I certainly don't believe that women should have to endure intense pain when there are methods to alleviate suffering and I'm not joining the conspiracy of silence that leaves women believing that it's all wonderful, hiding the bare facts from one another about the pain involved in giving birth (although I am aware it's a subjective experience). I believe women should know what they could experience and have positive and practical strategies for coping.

Since having children, the practice has been hard to maintain and it has been difficult to give it the energy it requires. Both my partner John and I often say we are just doing maintenance.

CHILDREN AND YOGA

Many parents and caregivers experience yoga's life-enhancing benefits firsthand through their own practices and so hope to give the same gift of yoga to their children. Children's yoga and parent/baby yoga classes are being offered to parents in some of the major yoga centers, but specifically children's Ashtanga is not. Both Guruji and his grandson, Sharath, advise against teaching children the Primary Series before the age of 12, for up until that age the body is in the process of developing. It is also true that a young child's spine will not be completely formed until the age of eight, so any adjustments may interfere with early development. A baby's spine is similar to that of a gorilla. The body is designed to crawl from side to side and the bottom tends to stick out. By the age of eight, the anatomy has changed to make the spine strong and upright. As long as no adjustments are made, showing children how to

do a given yoga posture is perfectly fine. Guruji and Sharath encourage children to "play" at yoga and to copy what adults are doing without being adjusted into asanas. This means that as long as there is an emphasis on play versus practice, it is fine to take your child to a kid's yoga class and let her enjoy the way her body stretches and moves into shape. As is the case for adults practicing Ashtanga, the body will "find" the correct posture over time and you will see that adjustments are a secondary influence.

As children approach the teen years they are exposed to many forms of stress. Yoga, with its emphasis on the concept of an individual journey and peace with yourself, can help children to meet their daily challenges.

Yoga teaches the individual to look within and to enjoy the body no matter what the shape. Through the physical achievement of yoga, teenagers will feel the sense of personal satisfaction that comes as their young bodies are able to do more. As a non-competitive path, yoga teaches how to get the best out of any body and therefore out of any situation. Everyone has strengths, and yoga works to enhance those strengths and to help with the aspects of practice or life that seem more difficult.

As a path of non-attachment, the essence of yoga is all about finding everything that you need within yourself.

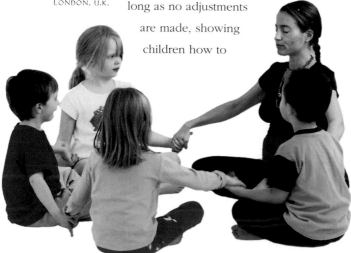

BELOW AND OPPOSITE: YOGA CLASSES FOR CHILDREN CAN START AT A VERY EARLY AGE. THESE FIVE-YEAR-OLDS ARE HAVING FUN AT TRIYOGA, LONDON, U.K.

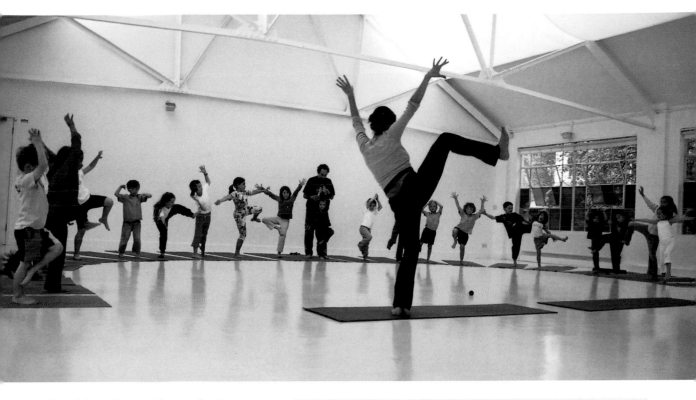

This philosophy provides a refreshing change from the habit of accumulating material objects to gain attention. Self-esteem and well-being are at the heart of the practice. In a culture where children are exposed to the media's constant messages of maintaining a perfect image and buying your way to beauty, the inherent teachings in the yogic path show girls how to find happiness within, not from "quick fix" methods. As for the boys, those who take up a yoga practice are often surprised by how powerful it is and how it enhances other sports activities, such as running.

In some schools, yoga is taught as part of the physical education curriculum thanks to the vision of some pioneering teachers, although this move is the exception rather than the rule.

PERSONAL ACCOUNT: ROBIN CATTO

Robin Catto is an experienced Ashtanga teacher and teaches yoga to children:

Kids can get into yoga very young. My one-year-old does a Downward Dog whenever he sees me doing my practice. Before they're crawling, you can do baby massage, which is like a cross between massage and passive yoga moves. This is excellent for loosening joints and creating good postural habits.

In terms of beginning a yoga class, four or five is a good age to start, because children are then able to understand that they are in a specific environment and are able to keep their attention focused long enough for some of the practice to be retained. At this age we use stories, games, and silly scenarios as a context for poses, primarily animal shapes and so on. By this age, children have begun to understand that what they are doing is good for them. Gradually, at about eight or nine years old, the child may prefer to be in a more "grown-up" situation where the teacher leads a complete class, taking into account the attention span of the group and not worrying too much about the form of the poses.

Teaching children is brilliant; kids love the fact that it uses their imagination in an unstructured way and they can then express that physically.

APPENDIX 1:
PREVENTING INJURIES

The Primary Series is known as Yoga Chikitsa, which means "yoga therapy." Each posture is safe and beneficial when the student and teacher work together intelligently without rushing. The following are key steps toward preventing injuries during practice:

BREATH: Breathing smoothly with awareness helps to calm the mind and to prevent strain in the body. Students working with the breath are less likely to throw or force themselves into postures.

BANDHA CONTROL: If the bandhas are used correctly the lower back will be supported.

ALIGNMENT: Good alignment can help prevent strain on the joints.

CONCENTRATION: When both student and teacher are concentrating on the practice, accidents are less likely to happen.

PATIENCE: It can be frustrating to see others working with ease while we struggle, but one of the best lessons of this practice is patience. It is better to work safely in the practice than to force yourself violently into postures and risk injury.

People do experience pain when they practice. Some of it is the normal ache of muscles and joints opening and aligning after years of inactivity. Old injuries may also reassert themselves, but in most cases the yoga practice itself will help the healing process.

Of course, accidents do happen. We do not always practice perfectly or focus perfectly and our egos can push us to work harder than we should. Here are some problem zones and advice on tackling them:

WEAK WRISTS: Create space in the wrist by standing on the hand as in Padahastasana (Hand-to-Foot Forward Bend), and pulling to stretch the wrist. If it is not possible to put pressure on the hands normally, it may help to bring the fingers together temporarily or rest the weight on the fists. Gradually increasing the work of the wrists can alleviate painful conditions such as RSI (repetitive strain injury).

SHOULDER PAIN: Women often hunch their shoulders up and in to protect the breasts. Over time, this position can cause alignment problems such as bursitis or frozen shoulder, which in turn may cause problems when working on jump-throughs or handstands. While practicing always keep the chest open and shoulders down and back. Shoulder injuries may also come from impact moves, such as jumping through. You may wish to see a sports injury massage therapist for deep tissue work or try acupuncture to help alleviate soft tissue pain.

LOWER BACK PAIN: If upper body strength is insufficient to lower the chin toward the floor in Chatturanga Dandasana (All Fours Staff), the student may inadvertently allow the hips to slump to the floor as support, thus pinching the lower back, which will be exaggerated in the transition to Upward Dog. If this happens, the modified version should be used until the arms are strong enough to support the posture properly. Care should also be taken to emphasize Uddiyana Bandha. Often lower back pain is experienced during Forward Bend or Bridge posture. Extreme back bends can cause fulcrum pressure, flattening the lumbar curve and putting pressure on the spine. Be aware that this can create disc problems. Evaluation by an osteopath and/or chiropractor is advisable in the case of acute back pain.

Those with stiff hamstrings should bend the knees in forward bends to release the back first. Anyone with a history of a prolapsed disc should consult a specialist prior to engaging in practice, as forward bends may pose a problem.

TORN HAMSTRING (OR OTHER MUSCLE): A torn muscle can take some time to heal but rest, ice, and sports injury massage can help. It is best to return to the practice as soon as possible since gentle stretching will prevent the scar tissue from shortening the muscle. A torn hamstring may be the result of excessive forward bends or leg raises with adjustments. If the hamstring has stretched into a hyperextension, this injury may take years to heal.

KNEE PAIN: Westerners tend to have stiff hips, but it is the weaker knee joint that will pay in pain. There are many causes for knee pain. See a sports injury specialist or osteopath and modify the practice if necessary to avoid extreme knee bends and Half-Bound Lotus Forward bends.

Michael Herne, a sports injury therapist who has worked with many Ashtangis, recommends the RICE method for treating injuries. RICE

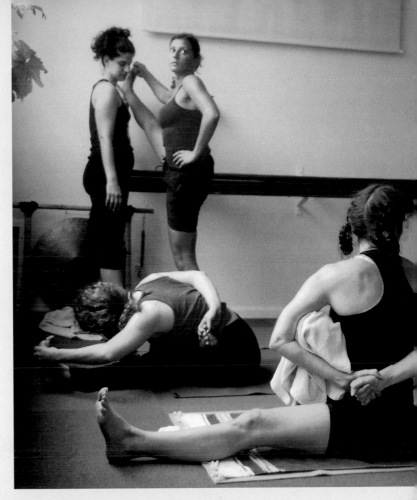

stands for Rest, Ice, Compression, and Elevation. When injured, your immediate response should be to rest and not use the injured limb. Apply ice (wrapped in a damp towel) to the injury. Bind the ice to the injury with pressure/compression. Keep the limb raised at a level higher than the heart. After RICE comes MICE, which adds Mobilization to the healing sequence. In order to prevent a limb from stiffening, it is important to move it gently. Again follow the ice, compression, and elevation sequence.

In general, preventing and dealing with injuries is common sense. Let your teacher know your weak points. Do not allow a teacher to adjust you if it feels wrong. If you do hurt yourself, use ice and compression to reduce inflammation if necessary, consult a professional, and then get back on the mat. Most injuries sustained in yoga can also be healed by yoga.

PROPER INSTRUCTION ON CORRECT ALIGNMENT FROM AN EXPERIENCED ASHTANGA TEACHER SHOULD PREVENT INJURY.

APPENDIX 2:
THE YOGA OF FOOD

See, I give you every seed-bearing plant that is upon all the earth, and every tree that has seed-bearing fruit; they shall be yours for food.

GENESIS

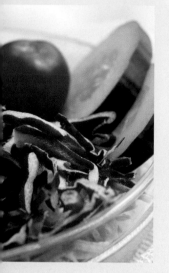

FRESH, RAW VEGETABLES ARE FULL OF VITAMINS AND ARE ESSENTIAL TO A HEALTHY, BALANCED DIET.

An important part of keeping the body and mind fit and healthy is the consumption of fresh, nutritious, and appetizing food. Anna yoga is a modern term based on the assumption that we are what we eat.

Originally, categories of food were related to the gunas, which in the yoga tradition are the three aspects or "strands" of reality and the building blocks of the physical world. All foods fall into one of these categories, either *sattvic*–"pure" and leading to serenity; *rajasic*–"active" and leading to energetic action, whether good or bad; or *tamasic*–"inert" and leading to delusion and ignorance.

Sattvic foods are mild tasting, easy to digest, and include cooked grains, legumes or pulses (peas, beans, and lentils), milk and ghee, fruits and mild juices, all consumed in moderation. These foods are said to appeal to those of an honorable and enlightened nature. Rajasic foods are more exciting and include garlic and onions; very sweet, salty, and spicy foods; and foods that stimulate the senses and encourage overeating. Rajasic people are more passionate and less controlled, with a tendency to be greedy and impulsive. Tamasic foods may include stale leftovers, unclean fare, or junk food, eaten greedily or without thought and leading to disease and addiction in the person who is drawn to them.

The ideal diet varies from person to person depending upon genetic tendencies and metabolism. For example, western cow's milk is processed and our wheat is much higher in

gluten than in many Developing World countries. These differences may account for the high incidence of lactose and gluten intolerance in developed countries. However, a vegetarian diet based on fresh, unadulterated whole fruits and vegetables, grains and legumes, sprouts and fresh juices, can form the basis of a healthy diet for most people. When you start with good quality organic ingredients, prepared simply and served fresh, and eaten in moderation, you are following a sattvic path to health and peace of mind.

Guruji suggests that people under forty years of age should eat two meals per day and those over forty only one meal per day. He also recommends that the stomach be one-half filled with food, one-quarter filled with water, and one-quarter left empty to allow for efficient digestion. Even healthy foods, when overeaten, become tamasic and difficult to digest.

Certain foods can be extremely helpful for conditions that affect women while other foods should be avoided. Here are a few recommendations:

Most women need more iron and iodine in their diet than do men, and these minerals are abundant in micro-algaes, such as spirulina, and seaweeds, which are widely available and can be added to smoothies and soups. Foods high in vitamin C, including vegetables such as cabbage, bell peppers, and broccoli, as well as citrus fruits and berries will aid in the absorption of iron. The bioflavonoids in these whole foods are also helpful in reducing excessive bleeding during menstruation and preventing varicose veins during menopause.

Ten days before the onset of menses, a woman's levels of calcium and zinc may decrease. When whole grains, legumes or pulses, and seeds are a regular part of the diet, this should not present a problem. Various seaweeds, green vegetables, and legumes are all good sources of calcium. Recent studies show that carbonated drinks (including sparkling mineral water) can leach calcium from the body. Since low levels of calcium can lead to osteoporosis, be sure to drink non-carbonated water.

Sufficient B vitamins, vitamin A, and proteins are normally provided by a good diet of whole grains, legumes, and colorful vegetables, as long as candy, alcoholic beverages, and junk food are avoided. Supplements should only be necessary if the diet has been inadequate for some time.

A very important group of nutrients is found in essential fatty acids (EFAs). Essential fatty acids are important to the whole body, especially the reproductive system, and also promote healthy youthful skin and hair. The easiest way to ensure sufficient EFAs in the diet is to take soaked or ground linseeds or cold pressed linseed oil on a daily basis. Other seeds and nuts are also helpful.

If you are trying to become pregnant, EFAs are even more important, as is vitamin B_{12}, which can either be taken as a supplement or consumed in seaweeds, algae, and nutritional yeast.

Women suffering from menstrual disorders should find that a whole food diet that includes the nutritional factors already mentioned, along with a regular Ashtanga yoga practice will help to regulate their cycle and ease any PMS symptoms or discomfort.

For a woman whose menstrual cycle has stopped (amenorrhea), Guruji has been known to prescribe a daily drink of saffron, buttermilk, and sugar. Often women stop having their periods when their body fat to weight ratio drops too low. If amenorrhea lasts longer than six months, it may cause osteoporosis, which is very risky when practicing Ashtanga and being adjusted on a regular basis. It may be useful to see a nutritionist. For most women, eating a little more quality food and adding good food fats to the diet will help.

Menopausal women have found that products high in phytoestrogens such as soy and linseed oil often ease menopausal symptoms. Taking vitamins E, B complex, C, A, and calcium can also help. Cutting out refined foods and avoiding stimulants such as sugar, coffee, and alcohol can stabilize blood sugar levels and prevent depression and mood swings.

Just as important as the food you eat is the way in which it is prepared and eaten. Guruji is very clear on the fact that food should be prepared fresh for every meal and his insistence is backed by his own youthfulness and the longevity of all of his family members. Taking time to prepare your food, sitting down to eat, and being relaxed and aware while eating will create a healthy relationship with food as well as aiding the digestive process.

Try not to be too strict with yourself, aiming for moderation rather than perfection, and think about substituting good foods for bad. To improve your practice of Ashtanga yoga, it is important to eat well because you are working hard. If you have a difficult relationship with food, don't worry—just keep doing your yoga and the clarity that the practice brings will help you to take food for what it is—fuel for a healthy body and peaceful and happy mind.

FOODS HIGH IN VITAMIN C AID IN THE ABSORPTION OF IRON AND CAN HELP REDUCE EXCESSIVE BLEEDING DURING MENSTRUATION.

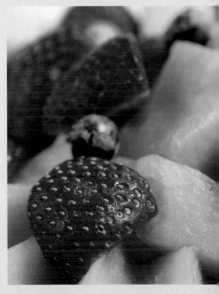

USEFUL INFORMATION

HOW TO FIND AN ASHTANGA YOGA TEACHER

If you want to start Ashtanga yoga, the best way to find a teacher is to go online and look at the links section of the key websites mentioned in this book. You can follow the links to an area near you and you can telephone to ask what is available. Some gyms now offer classes and this is a good way to check out how Ashtanga feels. At first it is fairly demanding but becomes easier with practice. Mysore self-practice is available only in cities or specific areas and so you need to make inquiries to see whether a particular center offers this form. Many centers will offer led classes; make sure you go to a beginners' class. Anyone can start at self-practice so don't think it is for advanced practitioners only. You will be taught the first posture and the rest will be added on as long as you can do them and remember what comes next. You have your whole life to learn The Primary Series, so take your time. The best teachers will have done self-practice at some time and you can always ask what their experience is.

Ashtanga Yoga Research Institute: *www.ayri.org*
Ashtanga Research Institute, #235 8th Cross, 3rd Stage, Gokulam, Mysore 570002, Karnataka, India.
Try the Ashtanga Yoga Research Institute for information about the founder of Ashtanga yoga, Guruji, and his grandson, Sharath Rangaswamy, the most advanced practitioner in the world, who together run the shala in Mysore. Includes information on how to go to Mysore to study Ashtanga self-practice. The site also includes information on world tours.

UNITED STATES OF AMERICA

Jivamukti Yoga Centers: *www.jivamuktiyoga.com*
Jivamukti Yoga Center Downtown, 404 Lafayette St, NY 10003 Tel: (800) 295-6814; Jivamukti Yoga Center Uptown, 853 Lexington Avenue, NY 10021 Tel: (212) 396-4200.
Jivamukti centers in New York offer Ashtanga morning practice, led classes, and the Jivamukti-style classes which include music, sequences, and spiritual discussion. The centers are wonderful places to find calm in the city.

Purple Yoga Hawaii: *www.purpleyoga.com*
Purple Yoga Hawaii, PO Box 29465, Honolulu, HI 96820-2645.
Run by the author's teacher, Cathy Louise Broda. She left to set up a center in Hawaii and is sadly missed in London. Cathy Louise and Glen run a dedicated center for Ashtangis and Shandor shadow-style yoga.

Eddie Stern: Eddie Stern, 430 Broome St, 2, NY 10013, Email: jaiganapati@aol.com Tel: (212) 431-3738.
Eddie runs morning practice in a beautiful central location in Manhattan and is one of the authentic teachers in Mysore-style Ashtanga.

Ashtanga Yoga Website: *www.ashtanga.com*.
A more general website dedicated to providing information and resources on Ashtanga yoga. The website includes lists of classes in the United States and the rest of the world and a number of interesting articles.

Yoga Journal: www.yogajournal.com
The *Yoga Journal* has covered a wide variety of styles of yoga for over a quarter of a century. This website complements the magazine by providing lots of useful information online.

UNITED KINGDOM

Astanga Yoga London: *www.astangayogalondon.com*
Astanga Yoga London, Diorama Arts Centre, 34 Osnaburgh Street, London NW1 3ND.
Hamish Hendry is certified by Guruji and runs the Astanga Yoga London center along with Roberta, Anna, and Denise. This is where Sally and Michaela practice and many of the visiting teachers come from Mysore. The links on this site can lead you to centers in London and all over Europe. Yoga holidays are also advertised.

Breathe: *www.breatheonline.com*
Classes meet at Triyoga (see below). Robin and Emma Catto are both Ashtanga teachers and they also teach yoga to children. This site offers a range of practitioners who teach yoga in your own home as well as alternative therapies such as massage.

The Life Centre: *www.thelifecentre.org*
15 Edge Street, London W8 7PN Tel: 020-7221-4602.
A West London Ashtanga yoga center that offers Lynne Pinette's pregnancy classes as well as Ashtanga classes.

John & Lucy Scott: *www.johnscottashtanga.co.uk*
5 Lafrowda Terrace, St Just, Penzance, Cornwall TR19 7LH. John and Lucy Scott are both Ashtanga teachers. John is certified by Guruji and offers workshops in London and around Britain and Europe. He is one of the foremost teachers and has published his own books as well as a DVD showing the Primary Series. Contact this site for many links, yoga products such as shiva mats, and yoga retreats.

Triyoga: *www.triyoga.co.uk* 6 Erskine Road, Primrose Hill, London NW3 3AJ Tel: 020-7483-3344.
Triyoga is a beautiful center in Primrose Hill, London. It offers self-practice and led Ashtanga classes as well as many other forms of yoga and alternative therapies. Triyoga also holds children's classes and pregnancy classes.

Michael Hearn, Sports Massage Therapist: Michael Hearn, 151 Whittington Rd, London N22 Tel: 020-8888-8699.

The Active Birth Centre: *www.activebirthcentre.com*
The Active Birth Centre, 25 Bickerton Rd, London N19 Tel: 020-7482-5554.

RESOURCES

Bender Birch, Beryl. *Power Yoga*. Prion, London, 1995. First published by Simon and Schuster, London, 1995.

Desikachar, TKV. *Patanjali's Yogasutras: An Introduction*. Affiliated East-West Press, New Delhi, 1987.

Eknath, Easwaran. *Bhagavad Gita*, Translation and Introduction. Arkana, London, 1985.

Elias, Jason and Ketcham, Katherine. *In the House of the Moon*. Hodder & Stoughton, London, 1996.

Feuerstein, Georg. *Shambhala Encyclopedia of Yoga, The*. Shambhala Publications, Boston, Mass., 1997.

Iyengar, BKS. *Light on the Yoga Sutras of Patanjali*. Thorsons (Aquarian Press), London, 1993.

Iyengar, BKS. *Light on Yoga*. Thorsons (Aquarian Press), London, 1991. First published by George Allen & Unwin, London, 1966, 1968, 1976.

Jois, Sri K Pattabhi. *Yoga Mala*. Eddie Stern/Patanjali Yoga Shala, New York 2000. First published in Canada, 1962.

Lino Miele. *Astanga Yoga*. International Federation of Astanga Yoga Centres.

Mehta, Silva, Mira and Shyam. *Yoga the Iyengar Way*. Alfred A Knopf, New York, 1996.

Pitchford, Paulm. *Healing with Whole Foods*. North Atlantic Books, Berkeley, California, 1993.

Ramaswami, Srivatsa. *Yoga for the Three Stages of Life*. Inner Traditions International, Rochester, Vermont, 2000.

Scott, John, *Ashtanga Yoga*. Gaia Books, London, 2000.

Shuttle, Penelope and Redgrove, Peter. *Wise Wound, The: Menstruation and Everywoman*. HarperCollins, London, 1994.

Sjomar N.E.. *Yoga Tradition of the Mysore Palace, The*. Abhinav Publications, New Delhi, 1996.

Additional Information from lectures, interviews, and private conversations with Sri K Pattabhi Jois, Sharath Rangaswamy, Saraswathi Rangaswamy, T.K.V. Desikachar, and numerous western yoga teachers.

INDEX

A

Ahimsa 17–18
All Fours Staff (Chatturanga Dandasana) 28
amenorrhea 115, 125
Anjusta ma dyai (drishti) 25
Anna yoga 124
Aparigraha 17, 18
Ardha Baddha Padma Paschimottanasana (Seated Half-bound Lotus Forward Bend) 66
Ardha Baddha Padmottanasana (Standing Half-bound Lotus Forward Bend) 54–5
asanas 16, 108
Ashtanga Vinyasa yoga 12–15
Ashteya 17, 18

B

babies and yoga 120
back pain 122–3
Baddha Konasana (Cobbler's Seat) 85
Baddha Padmasana (Bound Lotus) 104
Balance (Uth Phuthi) 105
bandhas 24–5
Benson, Herbert 116–17
Bent Knee Forward Bend A (Janu Sirsasana A) 68
Bent Knee Forward Bend B (Janu Sirsasana B) 69
Bent Knee Forward Bend C (Janu Sirsasana C) 70–1
Bhagavad Gita 10, 14
Bhakti yoga 11
Bhujapidasana (Shoulder Press) 78–9
Boat Posture (Navasana) 76–7
books 126
Bound Bridge (Setu Bandhasana) 92–3
Bound Lotus (Baddha Padmasana) 104
Bound Toe Forward Bend (Padangusthasana) 35
Bound Toe Seated Balance (Ubhaya Padangusthasana) 90
Brahmacharya 17, 18
Bramachari, Sri Ramamohan 12
breath 23–4
Breathing Sequence 104–5
Broomadhya (drishti) 25

C

Catto, Emma 118
Catto, Robin 121
Chatturanga Dandasana (All Fours Staff) 28
children and yoga 120–1
Cobbler's Seat (Baddha Konasana) 85

D

Dandasana (Staff Posture) 61
Desikachar, T.K.V. 18
Devi, Indra (Zhenia Labunskaia) 14–15
Dharana 17
Downward Dog 27, 28
Dristi 25

E

Ear Squeeze (Karnapidasana) 98
"eight limbs" 16–17

Extended Leg Balances (Utthita Hasta Padangusthasana) 52–3
Extended Triangle (Utthita Trikonasana) 38–9
Eyerman, Ken 109

F

Face Up Bow (Urdhva Dhanurasana) 94–5
Face Up Forward Bend (Urdhva Mukha Paschimottanasana) 91
Face Up Lotus (Urdhva Padmasana) 99
fertility 116–17, 125
Fetus in the Womb (Garbha Pindasana) 82–3
Fetus (Pindasana) 99
Finishing Sequence 96–105
Fish (Matsayasana) 100
food 124–5

G

Garbha Pindasana (Fetus in the Womb) 82–3
Goraksha 10, 11
Guruji (Sri Krishna Pattabhi Jois) 6, 7, 13–15, 18, 19, 25, 109, 112, 115, 120, 124, 125

H

Halasana (Plow) 98
hamstrings, torn 123
Hand-to-foot Forward Bend (Padahastasana) 36–7
Hastagrai (drishti) 25
Hatha yoga 11
Head Stand (Sirsasana) 102–3
Herne, Michael 123
history of yoga 10–11
Huxley, Aldous 10

I

infertility see fertility
injuries 122–3
Ireland, Derek 109
Ishvara pranidhana 19
Iyengar, B.K.S. 18
Iyengar, Geeta 115

J

Janu Sirsasana A (Bent Knee Forward Bend A) 68
Janu Sirsasana B (Bent Knee Forward Bend B) 69
Janu Sirsasana C (Bent Knee Forward Bend C) 70–1
Jnana yoga 11

K

Karma yoga 11
Karnapidasana (Ear Squeeze) 98
knee pain 123
Krishnamacharya, Tirumalai 12, 13, 14, 15
Kukkutasana (The Rooster) 84
Kurmasana (The Tortoise) 80

L

Labunskaia, Zhenia see Devi, Indra (Zhenia Labunskaia)
Lateral Extension (Utthita Parsvakonasana) 42–3

Lateral Forward Bend (Parsvottanasana) 50–1
Leg Extension (Uttanapadasana) 101
Linking Movements (Vinyasa) 64
lower back pain 122–3

M

Mangala Mantra 96
mantras 21, 23, 96
Marichyasana A (Posture of the Sage A) 72
Marichyasana B (Posture of the Sage B) 73
Marichyasana C (Posture of the Sage C) 74
Marichyasana D (Posture of the Sage D) 75
mats 22
Matsayasana (Fish) 100
menopause 108, 125
menstruation 6–7, 112–13, 114–15
problems 115, 125
moon 112–13, 114
Mula Bandha 24–5
muscles, torn 123

N

Nabi chakra (drishti) 25
Nasagrai (drishti) 25
Navasana (Boat Posture) 76–7
Neutral Pose (Samasthitih) 23
Niyama 16, 17, 19

O

osteoporosis 125
ovulation 112–13, 114

P

Padahastasana (Hand-to-foot Forward Bend) 36–7
Padangusthasana (Bound Toe Forward Bend) 35
Padhaioragrai (drishti) 25
pain 122–3
Parivrtta Parsvakonasana A-D (Revolving Lateral Extension) 44–5
Parivrtta Trikonasana (Revolving Triangle) 40–1
Parsva (drishti) 25
Parsvottanasana (Lateral Forward Bend) 50–1
Paschimottanasana (Seated Forward Bend) 62–3
Patanjali 12, 16
Pattabhi Jois, Sri Krishna see Guruji
Pindasana (Fetus) 99
Pinette, Lynne 109
Plow (Halasana) 98
PMS (premenstrual syndrome) 115
Posture of the Sage A (Marichyasana A) 72
Posture of the Sage B (Marichyasana B) 73
Posture of the Sage C (Marichyasana C) 74
Posture of the Sage D (Marichyasana D) 75
practice
preparations for 22
timing 22, 110–11
Pranayama 16
Prasarita Padottanasana (Wide-legged Forward Bend) 46–9

Pratayahara 17
pregnancy 6, 7, 118–19
premenstrual syndrome (PMS) 115
preparations for practice 22
Purvottanasana (Seated Back Bend) 65

R
Raja yoga 11
rajasic foods 124
Rangaswamy, Sharath 120
reincarnation 13
Relaxation 105
Revolving Lateral Extension (Parivrtta
    Parsvakonasana A–D) 44–5
Revolving Triangle (Parivrtta Trikonasana) 40–1
Rooster, The (Kukkutasana) 84
RSI (repetitive strain injury) 122

S
Sai yoga 15
Salamba Sarvangasana (Shoulder Stand) 97
Samadhi 17
Samasthedhi 111
Samasthitih (Neutral Pose) 23
Sankalpa 113
Santosha 19
sattvic foods 124
Satya 17, 18
Saucha 19
Scott, John 109
Scott, Lucy 109, 119
Seat of Power (Utkatasana) 56–7
Seated Angle Pose (Upavishta Konasana) 86
Seated Back Bend (Purvottanasana) 65
Seated Forward Bend (Paschimottanasana) 62–3
Seated Half-bound Lotus Forward Bend (Ardha Baddha
    Padma Paschimottanasana) 66
Setu Bandhasana (Bound Bridge) 92–3
shoulder pain 122
Shoulder Press (Bhujapidasana) 78–9
Shoulder Stand (Salamba Sarvangasana) 97
Sirsasana (Head Stand) 102–3
Sitting Postures 60–95

Sleeping Tortoise (Supta Kurmasana) 81
Staff Posture (Dandasana) 61
Standing Half-bound Lotus Forward Bend (Ardha Baddha
    Padmottanasana) 54–5
Standing Postures 34–55
sun 110–11
sun salutations 26, 110–11
Sun Salute A (Surya Namaskara A) 27–9
Sun Salute B (Surya Namaskara B) 30–3
Supine Angle Pose (Supta Konasana) 87
Supine Leg Raises (Supta Padangusthasana) 88–9
Supta Konasana (Supine Angle Pose) 87
Supta Kurmasana (Sleeping Tortoise) 81
Supta Padangusthasana (Supine Leg Raises) 88–9
Surya Namaskara A (Sun Salute A) 27–9
Surya Namaskara B (Sun Salute B) 30–3
Svadhyaya 19

T
tamasic foods 124
Tantrism 11
Tapas 19
teachers, finding 126
teenagers 120–1
timing of practice 22, 110–11
Tiriangmukhaikapada Paschimottanasana (Transverse Bent
    Knee Forward Bend) 67
Tortoise, The (Kurmasana) 80
Transverse Bent Knee Forward Bend (Tiriangmukhaikapada
    Paschimottanasana) 67

U
Ubhaya Padangusthasana (Bound Toe Seated Balance) 90
Uddiyana Bandha 25
Ujjayi breath 16, 24
Upavishta Konasana (Seated Angle Pose) 86
Upward Dog 27, 28
Urdhva Dhanurasana (Face Up Bow) 94–5
Urdhva (drishti) 25
Urdhva Mukha Paschimottanasana (Face Up Forward
    Bend) 91
Urdhva Padmasana (Face Up Lotus) 99
Uth Phuthi (Balance) 105

Utkatasana (Seat of Power) 56–7
Uttanapadasana (Leg Extension) 101
Utthita Hasta Padangusthasana (Extended Leg
    Balances) 52–3
Utthita Parsvakonasana (Lateral Extension) 42–3
Utthita Trikonasana (Extended Triangle) 38–9

V
Vinyasa (Linking Movements) 64
Vinyasa (term) 23
Virabhadrasana A and B (Warrior Postures) 58–9

W
Warrell, Radha 109
Warrior Postures (Virabhadrasana A and B) 58–9
Warrior Sequence 56–9
websites 126
Wide-legged Forward Bend (Prasarita Padottanasana) 46–9
women and yoga 6–7, 14–15
wrists, weak 122

Y
Yama 16, 17–18
Yoga Kuruntha 14
Yoga Pradipika 14
Yoga Sutras 14, 16
Yogarahasya 12

ACKNOWLEDGMENTS

Authors' dedication
We would like to thank Guruji, Sharath, and
all the Ashtangis who have inspired us and
a big thank you to everyone who contributed
to this book. We would also like to send love
to our parents.

Picture credits
© Krishnamacharya Yoga Mandiram: p.12; Corbis: p.15; Vanessa Fletcher: p19

Footnotes
[1] Devi, Indra. *Forever Young, Forever Healthy.* Prentice Hall Inc., 1953

[2], [3] Sparrowe, Linda. "Menstrual Essentials," *Yoga Journal* online, September/October 1999.
www.yogajournal.com/health

[4] Ramaswami, Srivatsa, *Yoga for the Three Stages of Life.* Inner Traditions International, 2000